BINGE EATING

10 Proven Unconventional Methods to End Binge Eating Disorders

SIMON GRANT & SOPHIA DURNER

Table of Contents

Introduction

Binge eating disorder doesn't just mean you tend to overeat once in a while. BED encompasses your life. You are constantly thinking about the last time you indulged and worrying about the next. Your physical health will suffer, but so will your mental health. It's now time to say goodbye to BED and begin a healthier life. Let's take the first step on the journey to a life free from BED and say goodbye to unhealthy eating habits!

Part One

Make Your Kitchen a Haven
for Healthy Eating

If you are reading this book, then you already know you are prone to bad eating habits. You may have already made attempts to fill your kitchen with foods that are seemingly good for you. But some foods are masquerading as healthy options that can completely throw your eating habits out of synch. We all know white rice and pasta are not ideal when you are trying to lose weight, but are there other staples that should be ditched?

First, we will find out what may be lurking in your pantry that needs to be ditched.

These are the foods that should be trashed immediately:

1) Cream-based products: On a cold winter evening, it can be comforting to curl up in front of the television with a hearty bowl of creamy soup. It will warm you up and fill you with hearty ingredients, right? Well, cream-based soups are just one of many foods filled with hydrolyzed proteins, unhealthy food dyes, and corn syrup. They are filled with empty calories and can also upset your stomach.

Similarly, creamy sauces may enhance a simple piece of chicken and make it seem tastier, but they are not a healthy option. Stay away from creamy pasta sauces and other unhealthy choices of sauce.

2) Baked goods: If you love to shop at your local bakery and cannot resist their tasty pastries and cakes, then you need to rethink your shopping strategies. Even the healthiest options could contain hydrogenated oils to extend the shelf life of their goods. These synthetically produced ingredients can increase your cholesterol levels and up your risk of a heart attack and stroke.

3) Fruit Smoothies: These products are often marketed as a healthy pick me up between meals. However, the truth is that most of these smoothies are more like a sugar-filled dessert than a healthy diet-friendly option. The smoothies are often packed with dairy bases and sweeteners that are high in calorific value.

4) Rice Cakes: Okay, we were all fooled by the humble rice cake. Seen as a healthy substitute for bread these diet staples are high on the glycemic index. Put simply; they consist of simple carbohydrates that provide a rush of energy when eaten but can leave you hungry after an hour or two. They are also responsible for triggering the craving area of the brain that can lead to binge eating.

5) Granola: Healthy looking and packed with protein, right? Granola looks like the breakfast of champions, but it is, in fact, one of the biggest health food imposters on the market! One small cup of granola has over 600 calories and contains 25 grams of sugar. You may as well have two pieces of fatty cheesecake for breakfast.

6) Processed foods: We could break down this category into different types of processed goods. However, the general rule of thumb you should be avoiding all processed foods. Deli meat may look healthy and tasty, but it contains chemicals and sugar. Pizza and bacon should also make the list of foods to avoid. Any food that has dextrose, maltose, and any type of trans fat should be assigned to the trash.

7) Low-fat foods: Surely low-fat options are better for you than full-fat versions of the same food? Well, the simple answer is no, not really. These items are packed with harmful chemicals that attempt to reproduce the original flavor of the food they are based on.

8) Ketchup: Surely, a squirt of ketchup on your food doesn't make it harmful, does it? Consider the facts. Just two tablespoons of ketchup contain 40 calories and 8 grams of sugar. High fructose syrup is also a major ingredient and has been credited with properties that increase the consumers' appetite and risks of binge eating.

9) Bread: This staple food may seem harmless, especially when it is whole meal or whole grain. No matter how you look at it, bread is simply unhealthy and is packed full ingredients that turn to sugar once it is eaten. This spikes insulin levels and promotes fat storage.

These insulin spikes will also lead you to crave more bread and lead to overeating.

10) Fruit Juice: Once considered a healthy start to the day, juices can be just as unhealthy as full-fat sodas. Once the fruit has been transformed into juice, the fiber element is stripped out. Whole fruit and veg become concentrated drinks packed with sugar.

11) Nutrition bars: Like granola, for years, dieters have been using energy or nutrition bars as a substitute for food. Marketed as healthy snacks, they are filled with sugar and high in calories. You may as well eat a candy bar for all the nutrition you will gain from these types of bars.

12) Vegetable oil: This staple part of most of our pantries has a special place on the list. All vegetable oils, including soy, sunflower, palm oil, and canola, have such a negative impact on the body they are considered as dangerous as cigarettes! The processing of these oils involves the use of carcinogens and solvents that are extremely detrimental to your health.

You also need to be aware of foods that contain vegetable oil as a standard ingredient:

- Nutella

- Dressings

- Processed cheeses

- Cookies

- Noodles

- Margarine

- Chocolate

- Store made dough

Of course, this list is not inclusive. You need to educate yourself about food, so if you are unsure of an item, then take a good look at the ingredients. If you see an ingredient, you are unsure of then use Google to check it out. There is no excuse for ignorance. We are in a better position than ever before to make sure we know exactly what goes into our bodies.

So, now we come to the good bit! Once you have stripped your kitchen of all the unhealthy food, it is time to begin a new healthy regime! Just think about your kitchen in the future. Packed with healthy snacks, fresh food, and wholesome ingredients.

First, we need to deal with packaged food. Ideally, you will only have fresh stuff, but in the real world, we need some backup. There are a few tricks to picking food that is packaged, so if you follow these tricks, you can make healthier choices.

How to read food labels:
- Be wary of a long list of ingredients: If you look at a food label and it has dozens of ingredients, then it is probably not a healthy option.

- Understand what the order of the ingredients means: Have you ever wondered why the list of ingredients is not alphabetical? That's because the order indicates the predominance of the ingredient in the food. The first few ingredients are predominantly what the food contains.

- Avoid high fructose corn syrup: If you see this list, then put the package back! This chemically produced sweetener is responsible for obesity and other related health issues.

- Buy food with high levels of fiber and protein: When it comes to picking snacks for in between meals, you need food that is going to make you feel full. High fiber counts and levels of proteins will help you feel satisfied until the next meal.

- Be aware of sugar levels: Sugar content comes in many forms, so you need to be aware of all types. Sugar is addictive and could be a major factor in binge eating, so avoid all types.

Here are just a few examples of sugar types found in packaged food

- Molasses

- Buttered syrup

- Cane crystals

- Caramel

- Carob

- Corn sweetener
- Dextrin or dextran
- Diastatic malt
- D-mannose
- Ethyl maltol
- Fructose
- Galactose
- HFCS
- Honey
- Lactose
- Maltodextrin
- Maltose
- Mannitol
- Panocha
- Refiners syrup
- Sorbitol
- Sorghum
- Treacle

Healthy Fat Burning Food to Supplement Your Diet

Food is not always your enemy. It can be your biggest ally in the fight to lose weight or even just get healthier. Ditch the idea of starving yourself and choose these super healthy foods to fill your kitchen with.

1) Oatmeal: If you used to eat granola or cereal for breakfast, you might miss having a hearty bowl of goodness to start your day. Oatmeal is a great way to kick start your day. It is filled with high fiber content to provide you with a slow burn until lunch.

2) Berries: Blueberries, especially, are a great addition to your diet. Packed with antioxidants and bursting with flavor, you can add these berries to your oatmeal to create a fruity breakfast fit for kings! Berries can also provide a sweet alternative to candy or other sweet treats.

3) Eggs: Scrambled, poached, fried, or baked eggs are a fantastic source of lean protein and choline, a fat-burning nutrient that helps you turn flab into energy. Eggs can be used for breakfast lunch or as a main dish. Hard-boiled, they are great with salads. Take a couple of hard-boiled eggs with you as a snack on the go.

4) Sun-dried tomatoes: When you have a jar of these bad boys in the pantry, you can turn bland dishes into a slice of Mediterranean cuisine. Tomatoes are packed with beta carotene and lycopene. These antioxidants will help you burn fat and make your food taste amazing. At only 5 calories each, they can also be a tasty snack that won't spoil your routine.

5) Quinoa: If you are missing rice or pasta as a filling addition to your meals, try this ancient grain as a tasty substitute. It provides vegetable protein and is linked to increased rates of metabolism. Quinoa can be eaten as a hot side dish to most meals or alone as a tasty starter. Try using it with fresh fruit for a filling dessert!

6) Coconut oil: We have already established that the oil you cook with can play a major part in determining how healthy your food is. Coconut oil is a dietary miracle. Studies have shown that just two tsps. a day can help fat burning and lead to reduced belly fat. Coconut oil is not just a healthy option; it also tastes amazing.

7) Greek Yogurt: This creamy pot of goodness is incredibly versatile. You can cook with it or use it as a stand-alone snack. Brimming with protein, it also contains vitamin D and calcium.

8) Cruciferous vegetables: Imagine eating something that is tasty and filling and burns more calories than it contains! Broccoli, cauliflower, sprouts, and cabbage are all found in this category of vegetables. Fill your fridge with these tasty sides and crunch your way to fitness.

9) Peanut butter: If you love your peanut butter, then you have some research to consider. You can choose healthy options like Smuckers natural or Justin's classic peanut butter while avoiding Peter Pan and Skippy branded peanut butter. Once more, it is all about the ingredients, choose a brand that has just two ingredients, peanuts, and a little salt. Avoiding the over-processed kinds of peanut butter will help you burn fat rather than store it.

10) Cottage cheese: If you get a serious case of the munchies before bedtime, this is the food for you. It is rich in casein protein that releases milk protein during sleep that will keep your stomach from rumbling.

Now we will consider some of the major food groups and show you what should be top of your shopping list.

Meats

Despite the trends toward vegetarianism and veganism, meat can be one of the most nutritious foods available. The rule of thumb is to choose the highest quality unprocessed meat you can afford and treat it with respect. Cook gently and retain the nutrients it contains.

Lean Beef

One of the best sources of protein available. Packed with nutrients, it also contains bioavailable iron.

Grass-Fed Steak

If you can source this type of steak, you will be cooking one of the best cuts of meat available. The grass-fed element adds omega 3 and conjugated linoleic acids to the meat that can decrease inflammation in the body.

Pork Tenderloin

Often disregarded as fatty meat that isn't healthy, pork is now regarded as a healthy alternative providing you choose the right cut.

Ask your butcher to cut you a fresh pork loin, and you will have a cut of meat that is lower in calories than a skinless chicken breast.

Chicken

Breast is best, but all chicken meat is considered a healthy addition to your diet. Even the fattier cuts are acceptable, providing they are served skinless.

Lamb

This tasty meat may seem like a fatty version of beef, but it can also be healthy. Eaten in moderation, it can be a healthy source of omega 3 fatty acids as most lambs are grass-fed.

Fish and Seafood

These types of food are both healthy and nutritious. They are also incredibly versatile and provide nutrients that most people are deficient in. The health benefits are also important. People who eat mainly fish and seafood have been found to live longer and have a lower risk of illness from heart disease, dementia, and depression.

Salmon

Fresh salmon is a great source of omega 3 and vitamin D. It can be cooked and served hot as a main dish, or it can be used cold for tasty snacks and starters. Tinned salmon is okay for a backup plan, but fresh tastes amazing.

Sardines

Another oily fish packed with nutrients. Small and tasty fish is a great way to improve your diet. When choosing canned sardines to be aware that the sauce they are packaged in could be a calorific nightmare. Choose sardines that are packed in light oil or brine.

Shellfish

Available in two forms, shellfish are described as shelled mollusks (for example, oysters or cockles) or crustaceans like crab, shrimp, or lobsters.

Tuna

Widely available and packed with protein tuna is a tasty way to include oily fish in your diet. Again, you should check the accompanying sauce for hidden nasties and make sure you choose low-mercury varieties.

Legumes

This is another example of a food group that has been demonized in the past. The main thing to remember about legumes is that preparation is key. They need to be soaked and prepared according to instructions. Once they are ready for cooking, they will provide another plant-based source of protein.

Green Beans

Also known as the common bean and string beans.

Kidney Beans

The staple part of any good chili, the kidney bean is full of fiber, vitamins, and minerals. However, it must be noted that if they aren't prepared properly, they are toxic.

Lentils

High in fiber and protein lentils are great in casseroles and stews.

Peanuts

One for the nerds here! Not a nut but actually a legume, the humble peanut is tasty and packed with antioxidants.

Dairy

Cheese

One of the tastiest additions to any refrigerator cheese can be used to enhance a meal or simply as a nutritional snack. Choosing the right cheese is important and below is a list of the healthiest cheeses on the market:

Mozzarella: Low in calories, high in probiotics this soft white cheese is usually made from buffalo or cows' milk. Add to tomatoes basil and balsamic vinegar for a traditional Caprese salad.

Blue cheese: If you can handle the distinctive taste, this cheese will reward you with a healthy dose of calcium. It also contains cultures from the mold Penicillium. It tastes great in a salad with pine nuts and apples.

Feta: Usually produced in Greece this creamy white cheese can sometimes be salty and sharp. If you choose feta made from goats' milk it will be milder.

Ricotta: This cheese is often referred to as a lighter form of cottage cheese. Its creamy texture makes it ideal for dips, and it also tastes great served with fresh fruit.

Whole Milk

Often considered an unhealthy option for people wanting to watch their weight, opinions have now changed. A portion of whole milk contains healthy fats, vitamins, and minerals. The calcium in whole milk will also aid bone development and prevent brittle bones.

Yogurt: We have already covered Greek yogurt, but any other plain variety will do. Stay away from flavored yogurts that contain artificial sweeteners.

Vegetables

The humble vegetable is calorie for calorie, the most concentrated source of nutrients. If you can incorporate them into your diet, you will soon see the benefits. There are too many varieties to list but here are some of the best on the market:

Asparagus: A tasty source of vitamin K. Try it with melted organic butter for a knockout side dish!

Carrots: Crunchy and tasty when raw, they are also delicious when cooked. Carrots can add a splash of color to your salads and can also provide fiber and vitamin K.

Celery: Refreshing and healthy celery can be used to add crunch to a salad or as a tasty addition to most soups.

Cucumber: Low in carbs and calories cucumbers are refreshing and tasty. They just need slicing and dicing and will provide you with nutrients like vitamin K.

Kale: It can be easy to dismiss kale consumption as a trendy fad. The truth is that it is high in fiber and vitamins and can add a satisfying crunch to your salads!

Lettuce: There are many varieties of lettuce on the market. Iceberg may be the one you are most familiar with but consider trying some of the following. Rocket, Batavia, Butter lettuce, Curly Endive, and Belgian endive. You may find new ways to get your lettuce fix!

Tubers

These are the foods that will fill you up. They originate from the storage organs of plants and can make a snack into a fulfilling meal.

Potatoes

Most people believe potatoes are a bad addition to your diet because they are filled with calories. Actually, potatoes are loaded with potassium and vitamin C, along with a host of other nutrients. Plain boiled potatoes are one of the best ways of filling yourself up when eating. Potatoes are not unhealthy, but they can be cooked in unhealthy ways.

Sweet Potatoes

Loaded with healthy antioxidants and nutrients, sweet potatoes are delicious and filling. The sweet orange flesh is perfect served alone or with a dash of seasoning.

Part Two

Rethink your Mindset

A healthy diet is not restricted to a certain time period. The word diet can be misleading. It implies that you are entering a period of restrictions, and once you have achieved your aim, you will return to "normal" eating habits. Presumably, then you begin eating the way that caused you to gain weight or binge eat in the first place.

When put like this, it really makes the whole dieting scenario seem ridiculous, right? Making major changes to your diet is completely different to going on a diet. It is also quite overwhelming. If you want to make your food healthy without giving up tasty foods, then you need to rethink your attitude.

Here are some ways to help you adjust unhealthy to healthy:

First, let's see how you can change your shopping habits

Shopping with a list: If you have already cleared your kitchen of unhealthy options, then chances are you will need a shopping trip. You may feel that shopping with a list is unnatural and makes you feel like a beginner, but that's exactly what you are. A novice healthy food shopper, and as such you need help. Prepare your list carefully considering the need for proteins, carbohydrates, and fats your body requires.

Impulse shopping is not your friend. You need to stick to your preplanned list and only buy healthier items. You can also save money as some of the most expensive items we buy are generally impulse buys.

Fruits: We now know that fruit is filled with sugar, and our fruit intake should be moderate. If you resist fruit juice and opt for whole fruit instead, you will ingest fewer calories and more fiber. Fresh fruit is also much tastier than canned varieties and makes a filling dessert.

Hydrate: We know keeping hydrated is important, but when you are in the store, those pesky sodas can look too good to pass up. Replace them with sparkling water or buy soda water and infuse it with fresh fruit. Sometimes it can be difficult to think of liquid calories the same way as we think about solid calories. One can of full-fat soda contains as many as 200 calories or the equivalent of 3 eggs or 2 servings of vegan beef!

Stay clear of diet foods: We have already learned that the word diet can be confusing. Diet foods are a whole new level of confusion! They have usually had their fat content drastically reduced, but the need to compensate for lost flavor can lead to some harmful additions. The addition of processed ingredients can make the product even more calorific than their full-fat counterparts! Try buying full-fat products in smaller quantities.

Snacks: sometimes, your body just cries out for a snack, and it can be hard to resist a salty chip or tasty cookie. Instead of ignoring your body, make sure you have some healthier snacks to hand. If you love chips and find it hard to find a substitute, try popcorn. As a whole grain, it is packed with nutrients and fiber. However, there can be a problem with commercial varieties that use high levels of sugar and salt to prepare their products. Try making your own or purchase air-popped varieties. Never buy the microwave brands as they can be less healthy than a bag of chips!

Try this simple stovetop recipe

Ingredients

3tbsps coconut oil

1/3 cup of high-quality corn kernels

Salt to taste

Method: Heat the oil in a thick bottomed pan on medium heat. Take 2 of the kernels and add to the pan and wait for them to pop. Once they have popped, add the rest of the kernels to the pan. Cover with a lid, remove from the heat and wait for 30 seconds. Return to the heat until the popping slows down. Remove from heat and empty popcorn into a wide bowl. Add salt.

How to Create the Perfect Healthy Shopping List

Fruit and Vegetables

Hitting the produce aisle can be daunting. Try and buy items that are in season and grown locally. They will be tasty and cost less. Here are a few choices with some interesting facts to help you choose.

Try a tropical treat: Bananas and apples are great, but try and expand your fruit choices with acai, guava, and papaya. They are colorful, tasty, and packed with nutrients.

Passion fruit: This fruit is rich in potassium and fiber. It can be eaten as a dessert or served as a side dish with chicken or fish. At only 16 calories per fruit, you can feel the passion of this fragrant fruit!

Mango: Originally from South Asia, mangoes are delicious with sweet and savory dishes. Simply peel and serve for a vitamin C and fiber-filled treat.

Strawberries: Packed with vitamin C and manganese strawberries are a great addition to your basket

Pineapple: Sweet and juicy pineapples contain bromelain that is a mixture of enzymes that improve your ability to digest protein.

Avocado: Unlike any other fruit, avocados are comprised mainly of natural healthy fats. Try them smashed for a creamy topping to get your fats, potassium, and magnesium levels up.

Cranberries: These super fruits are impressive and contain vitamin C, manganese, vitamin E, and copper.

Vegetables

Asparagus: Nutritious and delicious. It contains vitamins K1, A, and B1 and iron.

Bell peppers: technically a fruit, these colorful peppers will brighten up a salad or are deliciously roasted. They provide a significant amount of Vitamin C.

Cruciferous vegetables: Broccoli, cauliflower cabbage, kale, radish, and turnips are all great additions to your shopping. They provide a nutrient-dense side dish or can be served as a main.

Butternut Squash: High in vitamin A, these versatile veggies are great roasted or can make soup or porridge dishes.

Carrots: Another great source of vitamin A, it is important to cook carrots with a fat source to make the most of this fat-soluble vitamin. Raw carrots are tasty, but you will only digest 3% of the vitamin.

Eggplant: This is another vegetable best served roasted. Boiled eggplant is not a great dish!

Leeks: Delicious on their own most people like to cook with leeks. They provide flavor and nutrients to otherwise bland dishes.

Onions: Both red and yellow varieties provide phytonutrients.

Parsnips: These biennial plants are one of the most versatile vegetables around. Boiled, mashed, roasted, they are sweet and nutty and packed with vitamins.

Pumpkins: Try these delicious veggies for your source of beta carotene.

Spinach: Popeyes' favorite snack is high in nutrients and one of the healthiest veggies in the world.

Sweet potatoes: Packed with beta carotene and super tasty.

Tomatoes: This staple vegetable that is a fruit is a crucial culinary ingredient. Delicious in a salad, they're also a key part of Italian and *Indian food.*

Zucchini: If you are ditching pasta but miss having noodles as a side dish, try making zoodles with this tasty vegetable.

Dairy Products

Milk: Stores now stock an impressive list of kinds of milk, and the choice should be based on taste, added nutrients, and availability. Try almond milk or coconut milk for a pleasant change.

Yogurt: Avoid sweetened or flavored yogurt and try Greek for a creamy option. You can always add your own flavors at home.

Cheese: If you love a strong-flavored cheese then try parmesan or goat's cheese. You can use less without sacrificing taste.

Eggs: Choose pasture-raised eggs for a healthier option.

Butter: Full fat and pasture-raised are the best options. Avoid varieties that contain hydrogenated oils.

Flour

Almond flour: Low in carbs and slightly sweet in taste almond flour is a popular alternative to wheat flour.

Coconut flour: Produced from the dried and ground flesh of the coconut, this flour can provide a healthy way to make bread and desserts.

Canned Goods

Full fat coconut milk: Popular in Asian cuisine, coconut milk is a great ingredient for tasty sauces and curries.

Tomatoes: Canned tomatoes are a staple ingredient for all pantries

Sardines: Make sure the sauces are low in calorie and not filled with preservatives

Tuna or salmon: packed with water

Kidney beans: packed with fiber and great in chili

Canned fruits: Check they are packed in juice and not syrup

Soups: Choose low sodium options

Protein

Whole chicken: Choose this option for a versatile addition to your diet. Use the carcass and left-over meat to make soup

Fresh fish fillets: Trout, cod flounder hake or halibut are all great fish

Shellfish: crab, shrimp, mussels and other tasty seafood

Grass-fed beef

Lean pork

Ground turkey: A healthy alternative to ground beef

Vegetarian protein: tofu and Quorn

Grains

Quinoa

Amaranth

Farro

Barley

Rolled oats: stay away from sugary oatmeal and choose steel-cut or rolled oats

Corn tortillas: Great with chili and salad

Frozen Goods

Frozen fruit: Handy addition to the freezer and perfect for infusing water

Frozen greens: Spinach and kale are perfect additions to soups and stews

Frozen vegetables: If the fresh option isn't available then choose veggies that are not served in a sauce

Frozen yogurt

Frozen shrimp

Oils and Condiments

Olive oil: Choose the extra virgin brands

Avocado oil: Great for cooking with and contains omega 9 fatty acid

Coconut oil

Tahini: Just a tiny bit of this condiment will make your meal have a more Eastern feel

Mustard: Tangy or mild choose the heat or smoothness you prefer

Jarred capers and olives: The perfect way to perk up a salad

Salsa: Choose fresh options with healthy levels of tomatoes

Red wine vinegar: This Mediterranean condiment is a simple ingredient to dress your salad with. Packed with healthy compounds, it can also aid weight loss

Nuts and Nut Kinds of Butter

Having a choice of nuts will allow you to make your own nut butter when mixed with coconut oil. Choose from the following to make healthy spreads.

Almonds

Peanuts

Walnuts

Pistachios

Pumpkin seeds

Chia

Hemp seeds for a nutritious addition to yogurt and smoothies

Spices and Herbs

If you are new to fresh, healthy food, you may not realize how important a well-filled spice rack can be. These bad boys can turn your ordinary meal into a culinary masterpiece in seconds!

Turmeric

Chili flakes

Red pepper

Garlic granules

Nutmeg

Saffron

Ginger

Allspice

Lemongrass

Rosemary

Vanilla

Garam masala

Greektown

If you find that cooking fresh food has enhanced your interest in all things spicy, then check out thespicehouse.com for an utterly amazing range of spices to help you create your spicy specials!

Snacks

Often the most dreaded items of shopping for people trying to eat healthily. Chips and chocolate can cancel out our best efforts in a matter of minutes, so how can you snack healthily?

Try these healthier alternatives for snacking

Dark chocolate: If you have a sweet tooth, sometimes chocolate is the only way to meet your cravings. Choose high-quality dark chocolate in small bars to replace your normal candy bars

Dried fruits: Apple rings or mango slices are perfect for a small nibble of sweetness

Pickles: For a savory treat

Olives: Black or green

Hummus

Grass-fed beef or turkey jerky: Great source of protein but read the label carefully

Drinks

We have covered the right drinks to buy in our hydrating section. Water and herbal teas should be high on your list. If you do have to buy fruit juice, make sure it is 100% juice and free from nasty additives.

Shopping Tips

We have listed foods that are classed as whole foods. No processed food or ready-made meals are included. Of course, sometimes it is inevitable that other choices will have to be made if the time to prepare food isn't available. Make good choices initially, and forgive yourself if you fall into your old habits.

When you are shopping, begin in the produce aisle and work your way around the outer ring of the store before heading to the inner aisles. This way, you will have the fresh, colorful items in your trolley to remind yourself to keep your choices healthy!

Choose the highest quality organic, farm fed, and pasture-raised products you can afford. When shopping for fish, try to purchase wild-caught products. The money you are spending on higher quality items is an investment in your own health.

How to Eat Out Healthily

Eating healthily and avoiding binge eating is not just something we do at home. If you feel overwhelmed by the unhealthy options that eating out can mean, then follow these handy hints to enjoy social occasions without breaking your new regime.

Eating out, how to make it fun and healthy:

- Read the menu before you go: sometimes a menu will be so appealing before you know it you have made a bad choice. If you read the menu online, you can pick your food before you leave the house. This will avoid snap decisions that you may regret later.

- Check the Cooking methods: Most dishes will come with an indication of how they have been prepared. Healthy options will have been steamed, grilled, roasted, or poached. Unhealthy options may include fried, pan-fried, sautéed, or crispy. If in doubt, ask your server how the food has been cooked.

- Order before everyone else: Other people's choices can often influence us. If you haven't already chosen your food, then be the first in your group to order. This will avoid you being swayed by other people's choices.

- Make a healthy swap: If your chosen dish comes with a side that isn't as healthy as you want, then ask your server to replace it with a healthy option. Replacing fries with crunchy veggies will not just feel healthier; it will also be more filling!

- Stick with appetizers: If the restaurant you are eating at is renowned for its huge portions, try ordering two appetizers instead of a main.

- Sauces and dressings on the side: If your meal comes with a sauce or your salad is served with dressing, ask for them to be served separately. You will ensure your food is freshly prepared, and you can decide just how much you eat. Ranch dressing or creamy sauce can make a meal double in calories.

- Fill up on soup: Having a simple bowl of soup can stop you from eating too much of your main meal. It doesn't matter what soup you choose to provide you send back the breadbasket!

- Ask for a smaller plate: When you are eating from a shared platter, you can be unaware of the amount you are eating. Having a smaller plate will help you restrict your portion size as you notice how many times you reload your plate!

- Share your food: Many European countries encourage a shared dish. If you are dining with friends and there is a dish you want to try, ask if someone else will share your food and halve your consumption. If that option isn't available, ask the server if you can order a half portion instead. If all else fails, ask the waiter to place half your portion in a takeaway container to have the following day.

- Drink water instead of alcohol: When we drink alcohol with food, it can lower inhibitions and lead to bad choices. If you do want a glass of wine, then accompany it with a tumbler of water. Take alternate sips of both and halve your wine intake.

- Slow down your eating and chew thoroughly: Eating out is a treat, so why do so many of us act like it's a race? Slow down your consumption and enjoy every mouthful. Count the number of chews you make per mouthful and try putting your knife and fork on your plate as you eat.

- Finish your meal with a coffee: If you are serious about kicking your sugar rush, then skip dessert and order a coffee instead. Finish your meal with a quality ground coffee and avoid all those dessert related calories in style.

Where to Eat

If your normal routine is to eat out three times a week at burger joints or other fast food outlets, then it can be hard to eat healthily.

All that fried food and processed produce don't give you much choice. Try rethinking your options and choosing somewhere that supplies you with healthy options.

The choice between multiple visits to a cheaper fast food place or just one visit to a more expensive restaurant should be simple. Make the experience special and healthy. Freshly cooked healthy food tastes so much better than the fast foodstuff, so retrain your pallet to enjoy the finer things in life.

Higher-end eateries also appreciate the food they serve and understand that sometimes less is more. If you research gourmet food online, you will see the food is more delicate and less likely to look like a huge portion. Quality food is all about taste and texture.

Avoid all-you-can-eat buffets whenever possible. An unlimited supply of food can lead to serious overeating. If you are at an event where it is impossible to avoid buffets, then choose a smaller plate or load the one you have with 70% salad or vegetables.

Finally, if the occasion arises and you have been diligent for the rest of the week, then treat yourself to a portion of ice cream, or a bread roll, or a piece of cake. Whatever you like in a small portion will help you face the world with a smile.

Part Three

Hydration is More than Just Drinking Water

When you wake in the morning, do you drink water or reach for a pot of coffee? Yes, most of us love a cup of Joe to help us wake up but consider your nights' sleep. You have just spent hours asleep without hydrating yourself, yet you don't feel the need to when you wake.

Water is not just essential to quench your thirst; it also carries out important functions within your body. Even more important is the percentage of water that represents your body parts. You may not correlate the effects dehydration has on your eating habits, but now is the time to change this perception.

Understand How Much of Your Body is Made of Water

Most of us know that the renal system depends on water to function properly, but what about our other organs?

Skin: The biggest organ in our body is made of 80% water. Drinking water also helps flush out evil toxins and keep your skin glowing.

Bones: We all know calcium is good for bone density and try to include it in our diet. However, are you aware that bones are also 24% water?

Blood: Plasma is the fluid that keeps our body functioning. It is made up of 85% water and enables proteins, ions, hormones, and other life-giving cells to circulate.

Muscle: 75% of muscles are formed by water, and if you fail to hydrate them, you can cause serious muscle pain. Dehydration can decrease muscle strength and compromise your body.

Brain: This hugely important organ also is 75% water. Lack of water can lead to headaches, brain fog, anger, and headaches.

Lungs: Your respiratory system depends on water. The lungs are 90% formed by water.

Signs of Dehydration

Thirst is not the only symptom of dehydration. You should be aware that when your body is telling you to drink, it will trigger your thirst reaction. You don't need to sprint to a fountain and gulp gallons, but you do need to drink a glass of water fairly soon. However, if you are regularly missing out on the water, your body will display other symptoms.

Dry Mouth

Mild dehy1dration will cause you to experience a dry mouth and sometimes bad breath. Your body is unable to generate saliva, and your mouth will be uncomfortably dry. You may be tempted to grab a piece of gum, but you should ideally hydrate immediately.

Pungent Pee and Decrease in Volume

If your urine is dark and smelly, it can mean you are dehydrated. Clear urine that has a mild smell is an indication your body has sufficient water levels. As your pee becomes concentrated, it gets darker and smellier, a sure sign you should drink more water. Also, you should be peeing regularly to remove waste from your body.

If you are only urinating a couple of times a day, it means your renal system is underperforming. This, in turn, means you will encounter a build-up of waste in your system that can form kidney stones or worse!

Dry Skin

As we know, the skin needs water, and dehydration leads to patches of dry skin. Ditch the moisturizer that comes in a tub and reach for nature's moisturizer. Cold clear water will help your skin regain its natural glow.

Low Blood Pressure

Lack of water in your bloodstream will lead to your blood pressure dipping. This can cause dizziness and fainting. In severe cases, low blood pressure can prove life-threatening. Avoid hypertension by hydrating your body regularly.

Constipation

Water acts as a medium to flush out waste from your body. Your intestines require fluid to function properly. If you don't flush your waste, it can lead to constipation.

Fatigue and Headaches

Are you always feeling drained and lightheaded? Do you wake from sleep still feeling tired? You could be dehydrated. Headaches and dizziness can be caused by a lack of fluids in the body and should alert you to the problem.

Lack of Tears

Severe dehydration can lead to you losing the power to cry. If you are feeling sad, but the tears are refusing to flow, it may be time to hydrate.

Most of the symptoms can be resolved with hydration. However, if you are experiencing severe vomiting or regular fainting spells, seek medical attention.

How to Stay Hydrated Every Day

1) Carry a water bottle with you: Sometimes it can be easy to forget to drink water. When you are busy and occupied with other tasks, you can forget to keep track of the fluid you are drinking. It can be tempting to grab a stick of gum or mint if your mouth is dry and craving water. If you have a water bottle on hand, you will be more likely to take a drink.

Treat yourself to a personalized bottle from Etsy or Amazon. You can buy fashionable bottles to match your outfits! Make carrying a water bottle into a fashion statement and be the envy of your friends. Numerous companies are now recognizing that the water bottle can prove a great promotional giveaway. Check which companies are offering bottles free with your orders and choose them.

2) Homemade ice pops: Summer can be the perfect time to make your own ice pops. Store-bought options can be filled with additives and artificial sweeteners that can be harmful. Making your own pops mean you know exactly what is in your tasty treat. Use fresh fruit or vegetables added to water and blitzed in a blender to make your ice pops. Use a Popsicle mold to form your treats or even simple plastic cups. Pop a wooden handle in and place it in the freezer for 4 hours. You can use whatever ingredients you like, and a splash of coconut water will give you added electrolytes!

3) Sparkling water: If you know sodas are bad for you, but you miss the sensation a fizzy drink provides, then try sparkling water. If you are unsure which brand to choose, check out these examples:

Perrier: The market leader, as far as sparkling water goes. Established in 1863, this French brand is healthy and stylishly packaged. It comes in a variety of sizes and flavors, so you can choose your favorite. Try the breakfast blend that includes vitamin C or the detox option Ginger T Perrier.

Voss: If you are looking for an environmentally friendly product, this Norwegian brand is right for you. All the water has been certified for natural flavoring and genetic compliance. It comes in different flavors like lemon cucumber and tangerine lemongrass that are kosher. They also contain nutritious calcium and magnesium.

San Pellegrino: Hailing from Italy, this amazing sparkling water brand has been around for decades. They provide a reasonably priced quality product that looks stylish and easily recognizable.

Crystal Geyser: If you prefer your water to be strictly sourced in the US, then this is your product! Founded in 1990, it doesn't have the same pedigree as the imported water, but this doesn't reflect on the quality. The water is collected from natural springs in the alpine area of the US, and the company strives to pass on the benefits to local areas.

How to Get your Fluid Levels Higher

If you are experiencing dehydration and your moods are being affected, it can be uninspiring to grab a bottle of water. You need the inspiration to increase your fluid levels, and the good news is that even a cup of coffee will provide you with some level of hydration. Keeping hydrated doesn't have to be boring.

Here are some ideas to get your juices flowing!

Infuse your Own Water

If you don't like the idea of store-bought flavored water that could contain all manners of sugar and hidden calories, then make your own.

All infused water is made in the same way. Add your selected fruit and herbs to a pitcher or container and then cover with water. If you want a mild infusion, then leave the fruit whole or sliced. If you want a stronger flavor, then bruise or squash the fruit to release juices. Place in the refrigerator for at least 6 hours to chill thoroughly.

Flavored Water Tips

The longer the liquid is left to infuse the stronger the taste will be, or you can add extra fruit for a stronger taste

- Frozen fruit can be used for a more intense flavor

- When you reach the halfway mark in your pitcher, simply fill with more water. The flavor will be milder but still flavorsome

- The best tasting water will be after a day's infusion

- You can use tap water, bottled still water or sparkling water

- Citrus fruit will behave differently and can make the water taste bitter

- You can cook the fruit in water using a slow cooker or instant pot for extra tasty water

Try these combinations to find the flavors that you love

- Watermelon, basil and kiwi fruit

- Papaya, lime, and ginger

- Mint, lemon and cucumber detox water

- Passion fruit, pineapple, and rosemary

- Grapefruit, cucumber, and mint

- Lemon, lime and ginger detox water

- Jalapeno, basil, and orange for water with a kick

- Guava, lemon, and strawberry

- Cinnamon, apple, and ginger

- Mango, clove, and orange

Once you have refrigerated your water for 24 hours, remove the fruit and herbs. Your water will then last for up to four days. If you have any surplus, you can freeze it in ice cube trays. The cubes can then be used to add flavor to plain or sparkling water. You can also add them to cocktails and iced tea as a visually pleasing and healthy addition.

The benefits of fruit infused water are many. The detox versions can help you clear toxins from your system and help you feel fuller during the day. If you love soda, then try these healthy alternatives that are zero calories, gluten-free, low carb, keto, paleo, and vegan!

It is recommended that you drink 8 glasses of water per day. Try replacing them with tasty infused water, and this target seems less challenging.

Tasty Herbal Teas

Herbal teas have been around for centuries. They are available in a wide range of flavors and infusions to suit all pallets. They provide a great way to hydrate with a tasty hot drink, or they can be chilled and used as an alternative to water. This in itself is a great reason to drink herbal tea, but what healing properties do they contain?

Here are some popular herbal teas and the added properties they contain

Chamomile Tea

Commonly known for its calming effect, chamomile is often used as a sleep aid. Just two cups a day have been shown to aid sleep patterns and lessen waking up during the night. Chamomile is also believed to have anti-inflammatory properties and helps calm stomach problems.

The antioxidants found in chamomile tea are also linked with fighting certain types of cancer cells. More research is needed, but studies show that people who drink chamomile tea just 4 times a week are less likely to develop thyroid cancer than people who didn't drink the tea.

Chamomile is also packed full of flavones. These antioxidants are thought to potentially assist heart health and lower blood pressure.

The overall effect of drinking chamomile tea on the body is thought to be attributed to strengthening the immune system, so the bone and skin health see marked improvements.

Peppermint Tea

Possibly the most commonly used herbal teas worldwide. It is primarily used by people who wish to improve their digestive system while benefitting from the effect it has on indigestion, nausea, and stomach pain. Peppermint tea is refreshing and tasty, as well as being a natural remedy for digestion.

Ginger Tea

Most commonly used to relieve nausea in early pregnancy, ginger tea is also packed with healthy, disease-fighting antioxidants. When used to treat period pain, some women have described the ginger tea reduced pain as effectively as using ibuprofen.

Some studies have suggested that ginger tea may help people with diabetes and help with blood sugar control.

Hibiscus Tea

This pink-red tea is made from the colorful leaves of the hibiscus plant. It has a sharp, refreshing taste and can be enjoyed hot or cold. The tea contained traces of anti-viral properties and was believed to have been effective at fighting strains of bird flu. These properties were believed to help fight off other viral infections.

Hibiscus tea does come with a mild health warning. It is best to avoid the tea if you are taking any kind of diuretic medicine as they can interact with each other. Hibiscus tea also influences aspirin use as it shortens the beneficial effects.

This tea will help lower blood pressure and fight stress, but the warnings about aspirin and diuretic medicines should be heeded.

Echinacea Tea

While there is no cure for the common cold, this tea is thought to shorten the duration of a cold. Echinacea will boost your immune system and help you fight other viruses or infections. The warm herbal tea will bring relief to the scratchiest throat and soothes the stuffy nose. This welcoming, tasty tea is a useful addition to any pantry.

Green Tea

This type of tea is touted as one of the healthiest on the planet. It is packed with antioxidants and has various health benefits.

The healthy bioactive compounds in the tea can promote weight loss and aid fat burning. It helps to boost your metabolic rate and improve physical performance. The caffeine in the tea mobilizes fatty acids and transforms them into energy.

Green tea also contains catchetin compounds that have various protective effects on neurons. This is believed to lower the risk of dementia, Alzheimer's, and Parkinson's disease.

Lemon Balm Tea

Lemon balm tea has shown health benefits in different studies. It improves levels of enzymes that can protect the body from oxidative damage to cells. There is also evidence to suggest this tea can improve skin elasticity that typically lessens with age.

As with the infused water, you can blend your herbal teas. Add herbs and mix the leaves to create a tasty brew that is both healthy and personalized.

How to Make your Coffee Healthier

We all know how popular coffee is. When you wake up in the morning, the smell of freshly brewed coffee can be both comforting and delicious! Many experts will tell you that coffee is bad for you, and you should switch to a decaffeinated option. However, opinions are changing, and some experts are saying that coffee is one of the healthiest drinks around.

1. If you want to hydrate with your favorite java, then here are some ways to make sure it is the healthiest option available.

2. Do not load your coffee with sugar: Piling a whole bunch of sugar into your coffee can turn it into a sugary treat. Try cutting it out altogether and appreciating the subtle taste of your coffee without masking it with sweetness. If you can't get

used to coffee without sugar, then try a natural sweetener like Stevia.

3. Choose organic blends: Coffee beans are grown in varying ways. They can be sprayed with pesticides and chemicals that are potentially harmful to humans. It can be difficult to source the amount of pesticide used by various companies, and the contamination levels will vary. If the thought of chemicals worries you, then choose a high-quality organic brand.

4. Add cinnamon to your coffee: Cinnamon can lower blood glucose levels and cholesterol. It can also be helpful for people who are diabetic. Just a dash of cinnamon can turn a cup of coffee into a tasty spicy drink and provide health benefits.

5. Avoid low-fat creamers: Ideally, your coffee should be served black to appreciate the rich taste of the beans. If you can't do without a dash of milk or cream, then use the full-fat options. Nondairy or low-fat creamer may sound like a healthier option, but they are often highly processed and contain questionable ingredients. A dash of full-fat milk or cream will provide a healthy dose of calcium, and vitamin K. Choose milk or cream sourced from grass-fed cows for a healthy way to dilute your coffee.

6. Add cocoa to your coffee: If you love a café mocha or other chocolate-flavored coffee at your local coffee shop, why not try a homemade version. The café mocha you have in Starbucks is packed with sugar and sweeteners, so it is not

particularly healthy. When you make your version uses high-quality dark chocolate cocoa and leave the sugar out!

7. Use paper filters: If you brew your coffee in a cafetiere your drink will contain cafestol. This is a diterpene that can raise cholesterol levels in the bloodstream. If you are wary of ingredients that affect your cholesterol, then reducing the level is simple. Use a filter paper to brew your coffee and ensure you still benefit from the healthy antioxidants and caffeine.

8. No caffeine after 2 p.m.: Coffee is great for boosting your energy and helping you to stay awake when you are tired. These properties are helpful in the early part of the day, but they can also affect your sleep. If you drink coffee late in the day, you will still be feeling the effects when you go to bed. Set a time limit depending on when you hit the sack and allow at least 8 hours of coffee free time before bed. Switch to a decaf option or an herbal tea to give your body a chance to detox from caffeine and prepare for a good night's sleep.

The bottom line is that when you are trying to avoid binge eating, a drink can distract you from food and be beneficial to your health. If you crave a sweet snack, then substitute it with fruit infused water for a healthy boost of flavor.

Chapter Four

Understand What Your
Body is Telling You

If your body was a doctor, what would it be telling you? Would it be advocating binge eating or extreme dieting? No. And while your body may not have been to medical school, believe me, it has your best interests at heart when it comes to diet. You fuel your body with food, so your body craves the best food possible to run like a well-oiled machine.

"Normal" eating involves listening to the signals your body is giving you. You will know when you need nourishment and recognize the need for healthy food to fulfill those needs.

Have a Conversation with your Eating Disorder

Now for the difficult bit. You must stop your binge eating. Just like the end of a relationship with a partner, some harsh truths must be stated. Think about it. Your eating disorders have been by your side for many years, and it's time to kick them to the curb.

Try composing a letter similar to the one below:

Dear Binge Eating and other unhealthy eating disorders,

Hi, it's me. I know we have a long and intimate history behind us, but it really is time you moved on. I have spent years waking up with you, having you by my side, and going to sleep with you every day. Guess what! I've met somebody new, and you'd hate them. They are called good nutrition, and I think they're wonderful.

So, leave, before I kick your butt. You have overstayed your welcome, and I now need sanity in my life. And guess what! It is all you and not me. Underneath this confused, frustrated, and guilty exterior, I am well aware of what I need to do to get back on track.

I would love to say it's been a pleasure, but it hasn't so off you go! And don't let the door hit you on the ass as you leave!

Okay, so now you know you have taken the first step toward healthy eating, it's time to realize just how hard you have been on yourself in the past. That stops now. You are entering the era of self-compassion and kindness.

Are you your own worst critic? You may feel like everything you do needs scrutiny and criticism, and you are not afraid to dish it out. Do you feel that if you can't be honest with yourself, then who will be? Who will tell you to get your house in order if you can't tell yourself?

Now think about the ways you talk to yourself. For example, last time you overindulged at a party or home, how did you react? Did you mentally beat yourself up? Were you dismayed and disappointed with yourself?

Now step back and imagine being in a room with two people. One of them is saying to the other the statements you have just applied to yourself. How do you feel about the person giving the criticism? Asshole maybe? Bully definitely! So, is that who you want to be? How different would your life be if you showed yourself some self-compassion?

We can sometimes believe that the only way to achieve perfection is to scold ourselves for every mistake. However, if you are constantly telling yourself you aren't good enough, the more you will believe it.

The same now applies to your new food regime. So, what if you have a bad day and scoff down half a quart of ice cream? What about reminding yourself that the old you would have finished the whole quart and give yourself a high five for putting it back in the freezer? You will make mistakes, and you will mess up. Try giving yourself a break and recognizing what you have learned from your slip-ups.

When it comes to health and fitness, you need to realize that self-compassion is an ingredient that's just as important as carbs and proteins. You are not only changing your eating habits and improving your physique; you are building up your mental self and feeling better about yourself.

Now we have dealt with the inner narrative what else is our body telling us?

Fad diets tell you to ignore your body's narrative. When it is telling you to eat, it is trying to destroy all your good work. They encourage you to fight the hunger pangs and commit 100% to your new way of eating. Fad diets also come with strict rules, and if you deviate, then you are a failure! And we wonder where self-criticism comes from!

Well, here's good news. We are going to ditch strict regimes and adopt a healthier way of viewing food.

- Many fad diets advocate the following approaches to food:

- You need a set of rules to follow

- When to eat and what foods should be eaten and how they should be prepared

- Count every calorie and examine every food for healthy ingredients

- What foods to eat and what foods to banish

However, these diets rarely produce the results we need. Hence the word fad. Our bodies should be the guiding light when it comes to nutrition.

Educate Yourself About What your Body Needs

There are reasons we eat different food groups, and mostly we eat them because we are told to! We are expected to follow experts blindly into nutrition choices and very rarely question them. Knowledge is power, and once you understand what your body needs and why you will make more informed decisions.

There are three macronutrients your body needs to function. Protein, carbohydrates, and fats. The body has no way of producing these macronutrients, and therefore they must be obtained through diet.

Protein

The word proteus in Greek is the origin of the word protein. It means "first place" or "primary and gives a perfect indication of why protein is so important to good health.

Proteins resemble long chains. Each link of the chain is formed from the 20 amino acids that help form the thousands of proteins your body requires.

So, what do proteins do for your body?

Two words, growth, and maintenance. Your body will break down proteins at a normal daily rate depending on your health and activity levels. This is a normal function and nothing to worry about as long as you ingest the correct amounts of protein for normal functions. However, when the body is experiencing high levels of stress or injury, it is important to increase these levels. During illness, pregnancy, and other life-affecting periods, you need to raise protein levels within your diet.

Biochemical reactions. Some of our most important proteins are called enzymes. They produce reactions that are essential to keep your body functioning. They encourage the body to digest food correctly, muscles to work, blood to clot, and produce energy.

Act as messengers. Another important protein is hormones. They are grouped into 3 main categories: peptides, steroids, and amines.

These proteins govern the major areas of bodily functions like sex and sleep. They relay messages between the cells, tissues, and organs of the body

Provide structure: without certain proteins, our bodies will lack a certain healthy stiffness. Collagen, elastin, and keratin all provide the body with functioning elasticity and strength. They allow your body to stretch and then return to its natural shape.

Maintains PH levels: Proteins act as a buffering device to help the body maintain a constant PH level. Without them, the body would fail to function properly.

Balances fluids. If the protein levels in the body drop fluid from the blood will be forced into a cellular area of the body. This causes swelling or edema and can lead to serious illness and even death.

Creates antibodies. Imagine your body is a battlefield, and the antibodies are your soldiers. When illness or disease tries to attack you, the more soldiers you have, the more successful the fight will be for you. These fights also allow your body to form an immunity to certain diseases; once the fight has been won, your body will never forget it!

Transports nutrients. Proteins enable the body to spread nutrients and vitamins to reach the areas that need them. For example, they help carry oxygen from the lungs to your tissues.

Provides energy. Now, strictly speaking, your body should not be using proteins as energy as they have all these other functions to perform, but in the absence of carbs and fat, your body will turn to proteins. This explains why your body should not be restricted to certain types of food but a healthy combination of ingredients.

Carbohydrates

Carbohydrates provide fuel for the central nervous system. They are also important for brain function and energy for muscles. As we have discussed above, the body should be using protein to perform important functions, but when we limit our carb intake, we starve the body of fuel, and it turns to protein for energy.

Carbohydrates are classed as simple or complex.

Simple carbs contain just one or two sugars and can be found in fruit, dairy, and some vegetables. They are important for the body and provide fructose and lactose for basic functions. However, there are also simple carbs in foods that are bad for us and considered unhealthy. Candy and soda are two prime examples of foods that have no nutritional value and contain processed forms of sugar. These foods are referred to as containing empty calories. Your body is absorbing all the calories without any benefits from vitamins, fiber, or minerals.

Complex carbs are made from three or more sugars. These types of carbs take longer to break down in the body and release energy. Simple carbs provide the body with bursts of energy and relatively rapid energy sources.

How the Body Converts Carbs into Energy

Your body breaks down the carbs into sugars, and these are then absorbed by the small intestine. This enables the sugars to enter the bloodstream and progress to the liver. Now the sugars are converted to glucose that is then used by the body for basic functions and brain activity. If the body doesn't require the glucose immediately, the liver will store it for use in the future. If the storage reaches 2,000 calories the body, then converts the carbs to fat.

Good Carbs vs. Bad Carbs

We are all aware that carbs have been demonized by "food experts" and a lot of diets recommend cutting your intake. This can be dangerous and cause your body to turn to protein for energy. Understanding the difference between good and bad carbs will help you make informed decisions about your intake.

Here is a quick checklist to see if your carbs are good or bad

Good Carbs

- Low in calorific value

- Contain high levels of nutrients

- Have no refined ingredients

- Contain fiber

- Contain low levels of sodium

- Contain only traces of saturated fat, cholesterol, and trans fats

Bad Carbs

- Are high in calorific value

- Packed with refined ingredients

- Contain sugar and honey

- Has little or no nutritional values

- Contains high levels of sodium

Have high content-saturated fat, cholesterol, and trans fats

Benefits of Good Carbs

So, we have established that the right type of carbs is essential to your diet. They are necessary for your energy levels and work as fuel for the body, but what else do they bring to the party?

Mental health

Studies have shown that people on low carb and high-fat diets are prone to depression and anxiety while others on low-fat, high carb diets showed lower levels of anger and stress. This is attributed to carbohydrates increase the production of serotonin in the brain.

Carbs could also play a part in heightening other cognitive skills like memory, visual attention, and spatial skills. Studies showed that a healthy amount of carbs could contribute to improved mental health.

Nutrients

We all know the whole, unprocessed foods are a key part of your nutritional intake, but what about the carbs they contain? Consider the so-called superfoods that experts recommend because of their nutritional levels. Berries, crunchy vegetables, sweet potatoes, and greens all contain complex carbs.

Whole grains also provide complex carbs and are a great source of fiber and nutrients. It has also been discovered recently that whole grains also contain antioxidants that were previously thought to exist in fruits and vegetables.

What happens when the body doesn't get enough carbs?

In simple terms, a lack of carbs will cause problems for the body. Imagine depriving your vehicle of fuel. It ceases to function, and you can encounter major side effects. Without a regular supply of glucose, we know the body begins to absorb proteins, but what happens when this occurs? The central nervous system fails to function correctly, and you will become dizzy and fatigued. Your mental and physical state will be diminished, and you can lapse into a state called hypoglycemia. This condition will lead to feelings of hunger, excessive sweating, loss of consciousness, and in serious cases, can prove fatal.

When the body is forced to use protein for fuel, it can put excessive stress on the kidneys that lead to the production of painful byproducts like kidney stones.

Fats

The very name of this micronutrient sets some people's alarm bells ringing. Surely fats make you fat, or else why would they be called fats? Well, the truth is the body needs fat to function. They are an essential part of the diet and should be consumed daily. Good fats keep your body healthy and contribute to heart health, while bad fats fail to protect your heart and increase your risk of disease.

A Source of Energy

We have learned that carbs are our main source of energy, but good fats provide a backup source should your body run out of carbs. Fat forms a concentrated source of energy and should be limited to around 30% of your daily diet. It is high in calories, but that should not be the first consideration when considering what fats to eat.

Fats and Vitamins

Are you aware that some vitamins become redundant without the addition of fat in the system? A, D, E and K vitamins are all fat-soluble vitamins and will cease to work if you don't meet your daily fat intake. Low-fat diets run the risk of damage to vision, calcium absorption, and blood clotting function due to a lack of vitamins.

Regulating your Body Temperature

Adipose tissue helps keep your core temperature at a regular level. Fat cells form these tissues and form a protective barrier for key organs in the body. Without these fat levels, a sudden impact or movement could cause the organs in question to sustain damage.

Good Fats vs. Bad Fats

In the same way that some carbs are better for you than others, the same rule applies to fats. Research is still ongoing, but there is evidence that bad fats should be cut from your diet, and good fats should be embraced. It must be pointed out that eating too much of any type of fat will lead to weight gain.

Bad fats

The bad boys of the dietary world are saturated fats and trans fats. They are potentially harmful and should be avoided whenever possible. These types of fats are identifiable as solid at room temperature.

Trans fats should be cut completely, while saturated fats should be eaten sparingly.

Examples of trans fats

- Fried food including French fries, doughnuts and all deep-fried fast food
- Butter substitutes like margarine
- Cakes
- Pastries
- All processed foods

Any food that is cooked in hydrogenated vegetable oil should also be avoided. If you are eating out or buying fast food, make sure you ask what oil was used for cooking your food. You are perfectly entitled to know exactly what is in your food.

Some butter substitutes can provide you with a healthier option, and the key is to check the ingredients. Beware of hydrogenated ingredients and products that claim to have zero levels of trans fats. Ignore the marketing and read the ingredients list.

Saturated Fats

These fats can be eaten sparingly and are mainly contained in animal and dairy products.

- Sources include

- Fatty meat products like pork and lamb

- Chicken skin

- Milk, butter, cheese, ice cream

- Vegetable shortening like lard

Good Fats

Food experts consider these heart-healthy fats to be essential to a regular diet. Monosaturated and polyunsaturated fats are good choices for a healthy diet. These types of fats are generally liquid at room temperature.

Monosaturated fats are found in a variety of foods and oils that improve your cholesterol levels. They can also decrease your chances of suffering from cardiovascular problems.

These foods include

1. Healthy oils like canola, extra virgin olive oil, avocado oil, safflower oil, and peanut oil

2. Healthy kinds of butter like unprocessed peanut butter and almond butter

3. Avocados

Polyunsaturated Fats

These are the essential fats that the body can't function without. They are only available from dietary sources, and this includes plant-based foods and oils. These fats are packed with two major fatty acids known as omega 3 and omega 6, which are essential for healthy living.

Find these fats in the following foods:

- Oily fish like salmon, sardines, mackerel, and tuna
- Oysters
- Anchovies
- Caviar
- Flax seeds
- Chia seeds
- Walnuts
- Soybeans

The bottom line to protein, carb, and fat intake is awareness. You may be aware that fried fast food is not healthy and should be avoided, but sometimes products labeled as "healthy" can contain hidden dangers. Food is essential to fuel the body, but putting the wrong fuel into your body can cause problems.

Part Five

Engage in Positive Self Talk

It is not uncommon for us to have a running dialogue dictating our lives. This is often referred to as self-talk. Sometimes the reason we binge eat is an attempt to silence this inner voice. Self-talk is the narrative that governs how you think about yourself. If your self-talk is negative, then it becomes essential for you to silence it.

What if we take another look at the narrative and encourage it instead of silencing it? Did you know your brain is hard-wired to remember the negative aspects of your self-talk more than the positive aspects? We remember when we do not get it right more vividly than we remember when things went great. Replaying the negative experiences helps reinforce low feelings of self-esteem that can then trigger binge eating.

How to Turn on the Positive Self-Talk to Break Bad Habits

As you may have guessed, positive self-talk is the flip side of negative self-talk. It is primarily about changing the narrative to your life. It is not about self-delusion or deceit. We are not encouraging inaccuracy in how you see yourself; we are just striving for self-compassion. You are carrying a negative image of yourself based on former disappointments. It is now time to change that image and forgive your past mistakes.

Positive self-talk can also help you reduce stress and help you to deal with stressful decisions positively. It changes your inner voice to "I can do this" or, in the case of binge eating, "I don't need to do this." You will also feel more confident and resilient. Optimism will replace pessimism as you change the attitude, and you will believe in yourself. You will know your goals, and more importantly, you will believe you can achieve them.

Positive Self-Talk Statements to Try

As an individual, you will know what triggers your negativity. In the same respect, you will also know what will trigger your positivity. Not everyone's self-talk will be the same, and only you can recognize the approach that works for you.

Here are some general statements that you can personalize to suit your needs:

1) I am perfectly capable of changing my mind.

2) I have the power to divert my thoughts away from eating and focus on other activities.

3) I will give my all to make this work.

4) When I master this, I will become a better person.

5) Today is the first day of the rest of my life.

6) I have the strength to do this.

7) This is just the first step on a long journey, but it is the most important one.

8) Even when I face a setback, I will congratulate myself for getting that far.

9) Food is not the focus of my thoughts; I have other things to consider.

10) Even though today was tough, I survived it, and tomorrow will be easier.

Understand What Triggers your Negative Self-Talk

How often do you have negative thoughts about yourself or the situations you find yourself in? Twice a day, a couple of times more, perhaps? Chances are you are unaware of just how many times you indulge in negative self-talk. Once you understand the magnitude of your negativity, you can begin to retrain your mind.

Negative self-talk generally falls into one of the following categories:

Personalizing: This is when your thoughts turn to self-blame. You feel you are the sole source of all that has gone wrong.

Polarizing: You fail to see any grey areas. Things are either right or wrong. The middle ground is an area you are unaware of.

Magnifying: You elevate the negative aspects of life and dismiss any positive elements.

Catastrophizing: You expect the worse. There is no room in your thinking for positivity.

When you have a negative thought, it is important to realize which one of these categories apply. This is the first step to reorganizing your thoughts and switching them to positive frames.

How to Switch Gears when Utilizing Self-Talk

Once you have recognized your triggers and categories, it is time to reframe negative phrases with positive affirmations.

Try these exercises to help you think differently. Take negative statements and turn them around.

For example

Negative self-talk: "I am such a failure; I finished that whole pack of cookies and two bags of chips."

Turn this around to:

Positive self-talk: "Okay, so I ate a pack of cookies and two bags of chips. It could have been worse. I could have eaten the other cookies in the kitchen. I then stopped eating and went for a walk. I am well on the way to kicking this habit."

Negative self-talk: "Why should I go out to a friend's house? My home is more comfortable, and I can eat what I like."

Turn around to

Positive self-talk: "Going to a friend's house will distract me from eating, and I will have a great time chatting with them. I am a good company, and I may even meet some new friends today."

The Imaginary Friend Exercise

Sometimes we think things about ourselves that are deeply disturbing. We believe the thoughts because we have such low opinions of ourselves. This exercise is designed to get some perspective on the negative thoughts we have.

Take a piece of paper or open a file on the computer. Identify all the phrases or comments you think when you have negative self-talk. Be honest and list the most derogatory comments you have ever thought.

- Once you have the list, ask yourself the following questions:

- Would any of your friends make this comment about you?

- Would I ever make this statement about a friend or member of my family?

- What would my friends and family say about me instead?

- How would I react to a friend or family member who believed this statement was true about them?

Once you study your answers, the truth should be identifiable. If your friends and family would not say these negative things about you, then why do you think them? If the thought of assigning any of the negative phrases to others horrifies you, then why do you assign them to yourself?

Make a note of the most recurring phrases in your phone or a notebook and replace them with positive examples. When you feel yourself slipping into a negative frame of mind, then refer to your notes. This will not happen overnight, and it will take effort. You are changing your inner narrative, and this is challenging.

Create a Self-Esteem Worksheet

Worksheets are a great tool when you are trying to change your habits. There is a positive aspect of seeing something solid every morning. Worksheets will help you focus your thoughts and give you goals for the day. Behavioral changes can be difficult to implement, but these prompts help you regroup and understand exactly why you are making the changes.

The ideas below are not just based on binge eating prompts. The idea is that improving your overall self-esteem will help you address the reasons behind your eating habits. These prompts are designed to help you celebrate different aspects of your life and deflect from your eating patterns.

Try these daily prompts to encourage positive self-talk:

Section 1:

I was proud of myself today because of I ….

I enjoyed myself today when I ….

I was happy today because of I….

Section 2:

My friends think I am great because…

The best part about today was…

My family loves me because I can…

Section 3:

I am really good at it…

I have some unique skills…

My best characteristic is….

Section 4:

I am looking forward to it…

I am planning on learning….

I am at my best when I am …

Section 5:

I was successful this week because of I …

My life is amazing because…….

My 5 favorite things to do are….

Make it Happen

Negative self-talk can often lead to you missing out on opportunities and new situations. The fear of what may happen prevents you from undertaking anything that is out of your comfort zone. That is when we are most likely to experience self-loathing and reach for food to make us feel better.

Realizing what the worst-case scenario is can be daunting. Your imagination can wreak havoc and lead to you imagining doom and gloom at every turn. Worksheets can help you curb those feelings and realize that the world can be a positive place. When the little voices in your head are telling you that life is tough, and you do not have the strength to survive, it is time to fight back!

Positive Examples Worksheet

This exercise helps you realize your worst fears and replace them with positive messages. It also helps you consider the emotions that accompany your fears and expectations.

Consider these classic situations that can appear terrifying and how to overcome them:

1) The situation is meeting someone for the first time.

The negative self-talk is: "Why would they be interested in me? I am dull and uninteresting. They will probably be bored."

The positive self-talk is: "I am interested and have a lot to offer to the conversation. This could be a new friend for me; I am looking forward to this."

The emotions should change from frightened and wary of excited and enthusiastic.

2) The situation is giving a presentation at work.

The negative self-talk is: "I will be dull and misinformed. They would rather hear this presentation by someone else. I may even lose my job; it is so bad."

The positive self-talk is: "Wow, I know my stuff. They are going to be so interested in what I have to say. I may even get a promotion based on this presentation."

3) The situation is asking someone for a date.

The negative self-talk is: "They are too attractive for me to even talk to; how can I ask them on a date? What if they reject me, and I am left looking humiliated?"

The positive self-talk is: "I like this person, and they like me, why shouldn't I ask them on a date? We are going to have such a great time together, and even if they say no, we can stay friends."

4) The situation is trying a new hairstyle.

The negative self-talk is: "What if I look ridiculous. I will not be able to leave the house, and all my friends will laugh at me. I think I'll stick to my old style and not risk the ridicule."

The positive self-talk is: "My new hairstyle will make me look so different. I deserve a new look as I am rocking my life at the moment. I trust my stylist will not make me look bad. Bring it on!"

5) The situation is learning an instrument.

The negative self-talk is: "There is no way I have the skills to learn an instrument. I am tone deaf and have stubby fingers."

The positive self-talk is: "I am looking forward to playing my new instrument for friends and family soon. Carnegie Hall, here I come!"

How to Make your Surroundings Help you Change your Mindset

Changing your inner self-talk is a battle that is fought on many levels. If you are in a situation when you feel anxious, you can revert to old habits quickly. The best way to stop this happening is to make your surroundings as positive as possible.

If you love to see positive affirmations in your personal space, then you are in luck! Current trends in wall hangings and soft fabrics are filled with cool messages and strong affirmations that look great hanging from the wall or adorning a chair! Choose messages that lift your spirits and fill you with hope. Visit Etsy or Zazzle to purchase your affirmative wall art or décor or just use the designs for inspiration!

Sometimes a quote can work even better than random phrases. If you have a favorite quote or piece of text, why not turn it into a piece of art? Maybe a piece of jewelry or a placemat.

The options are endless. Here are a few ideas to help you get started:

1) Pebbles: We all have access to stones or pebbles, so this could be a great start for beginners. Take some pebbles or stones and paint them with acrylic paint. Now write some affirmative phrases on each one.

2) Silhouette Art: Take an image of yourself with a sideways view. Trace the outline onto white paper and then cut out the shape. Place on a black background to create a silhouette of yourself. Take different colored sharpies and write your affirmations in the white image.

3) The Daisy Effect: On a square black background, draw a circle in the center. Use light paper oval shapes to form petals like a daisy that surrounds the center circle. Use sharpies to write positive sentences on each petal. Frame and hang on the wall.

4) Placemats: Take a pack of plain white paper placemats and decorate them with positive affirmations. You can choose large mats for plates or smaller versions for glasses and cups. Try taking them with you when you eat out or go for a coffee. You can leave them there to inspire others.

5) Jewelry: Take a simple round metal disc and paint them with acrylic paint. Write your affirmation on the disc and then pierce a hole in the top. Thread the disc onto a chain and wear it around your neck.

Here are some positive statements to put on your artwork:

- o   I can do hard things

- o   I am loving, joyful, respectful, faithful, worthy, patient, strong, kind, joyful, or confident.

- o   It is okay to feel feelings

- o   Problems challenge me to become a better person

- o   Dream Big

- o   Create Peace

- o   You are so brave

- o   I am loved

- o   You are precious

- o   You are safe

- o   You are enough

- o   Smile and the world will smile back

Create a Short Story Exercise

If you feel the negativity crowding you and cannot find inspiration in the real world, it may be time to try this exercise. Fiction can take you to a world where everything is dictated by your imagination. You can create a utopian world where you are the best version of yourself. You can try this method in times of negativity or bad thoughts.

Once you find the negative thoughts dictating your mindset, just stop. Tell yourself a story about a future in which you are achieving your desires and fulfilling your goals. You can do this mentally, or you can commit the story to paper. Create a version of yourself where you have control and restraint over food.

Once you have mastered this technique, you can use it to lift yourself out of any bad situations in the future. You will become adept at expecting good things to happen. Once you adopt this positive attitude, your personal circumstances will improve.

You can also use this exercise to take you away from the negative mindset completely. If you feel the situation is so out of hand that positive affirmations are not enough, then take your focus elsewhere. Maybe you are in a position of financial stress, and you feel the urge to compensate with food. Instead of fighting your thoughts about finances, try telling a story about something else.

Once you have distracted yourself with pleasant imaginings, you will find the urge to binge recede. You know the financial issues will still need addressing, but you will be in a better frame of mind. Imagine a holiday or pleasant day out in the future and picture yourself relaxing. You will soon feel the sun on your face, and the feeling of peace and relaxation will ease your stress.

What else can you do to improve your inner narrative?

Positive self-talk will take time, but you are now on the right path. There are a few tips you can try to help you on your journey.

Here are some of the more useful tips:

Surround yourself with positive people: We are all influenced by the company we keep. The outlook and emotions of your friends and co-workers will inadvertently affect your own moods. Surround yourself with people who are successful and positive, and their outlook will soon become yours!

Find humor: If you are feeling stressed and negative, think of an alternative way to feel better. Distract yourself with things that make you laugh. It can be an amusing cat video on YouTube or an episode of your favorite television comedy. Whatever your choice, make sure it is entertaining and will release tension.

Check-in with your feelings: It can feel self-indulgent to check in with yourself, yet we do it with our friends. If we feel someone is having emotional difficulties, we make sure we are there for them. Why not do the same for you? Take the time to ask, "Are you okay" and give yourself an honest answer. If you need it to give yourself an emotional hug or ask for one from a friend. We all need help, but sometimes it can be difficult to ask for it.

Part Six

Exercise for People Who Hate Exercise

Okay, so we now have a kitchen that is a haven of healthiness, and all the toxic snacks have been removed. Binge eating is now a thing of the past, right? Well, if only it was that simple. Your bad habits have been with you for years, and despite your best efforts, they need to be replaced with some form of distraction.

Now, before you consider skipping this section because you hate exercise, wait a second and consider how important any form of exercise is. We know that 90% of the battle is nutrition, but exercise should form at least some of the remaining 10%. Also, exercise and movement can be a great way to distract you from eating. But exercise sucks, right? Strength training, dumbbells, treadmills, and spin classes are not the only way to burn calories and stay active.

So, forget about squats, lunges, and hitting the gym; it's time to consider other forms of exercise. If you could burn just 300 calories a day, it would make a huge difference to your life. Sounds good, right?

Here is a fact that will blow your mind! Fidgeting and shuffling your feet for two hours a day could equate to burning 350 calories a day! Sitting still should be a thing of the past. If you are watching a film on the television, try pausing it every fifteen minutes and taking a 5-minute pace around the room. Even when you are sitting down, try air drumming and shuffling your feet to a tune in your head.

Now you get the idea! Ditch the idea of the optimal workout and choose some of these fun activities to get your adrenaline pumping while having some fun.

1) Walking: Okay, not really an activity that will light any fires in the imagination, but it is a classic example of the simplicity of the exercise. If you are restricted to the office or the home for any reason, then try walking around the room when you are on the telephone or having an online meeting. It was good enough for Steve Jobs, so it should be good enough for us!

If you want to take a less traditional type of approach to walking, try Nordic walking instead. Use poles to coordinate your steps and give yourself a full-body workout. This full-body exercise is easy on the joints and is suitable for all ages. You can embrace the experience with some sort of Nordic headwear, but it isn't essential!

2) Dancing: When was the last time you hit the dancefloor and let it all hang out? Well, the good news is that dancing can be done in the privacy of your home and can burn calories at an amazing rate! Think of Carlton in the Fresh Prince of Belair dancing to Tom Jones, and you get the picture. Next time you feel like raiding the fridge turn on your iPad and hit shuffle. Turn up the volume and let yourself go. You will soon forget about eating!

If you want a more organized dance experience, sign up for Zumba or Salsa classes. Maybe Flamenco is more up your street. Whatever form you choose, you will be exercising and having fun!

If you have kids create an impromptu dance session. Disney films are a great source of kickass tunes to dance to. As the lady said, "Let it go; let it go."

3) Create an obstacle course: If you are lucky enough to have space consider your obstacle course. Make tunnels to crawl through and balance beams to cross. You can use ropes to make swings and logs to balance on. All it takes is space and a bit of imagination. Household objects can be used to create tricky obstacles that are fun to conquer.

4) Bike it: If you have a boring commute to work, then consider swapping the car for a more challenging vehicle. A bike will get you from A to B while burning energy, saving money on gas, and helping the environment. Use your bike to visit friends and get those leg muscles pumping.

You may want to take it to another level and join a cycling club. Check local press or online sources to find a club in your area.

5) Ditch the elevator: When you enter a building that has an elevator next to the stairs, are you more inclined to take the stairs?

Of course, you aren't, and not many of us would. This simple choice can make a world of difference to your fitness levels. Taking the stairs will make you breathless for the first couple of times, but it gets better. You will soon be leaping up staircases and ignoring those claustrophobic elevators.

6) Alternative seating: Do you spend a lot of time on your laptop or seated at a desk? Maybe you are required to remain seated for long periods. Try squatting instead of conventional sitting. Our bodies are meant to squat, ask anybody who has been on holiday to India or Eastern Europe, and had to use the loo! Giving birth is easier and more natural when squatting, so try and listen to your body. Grab a book and bend your legs as far as possible. Remain squatted for fifteen minutes and feel the benefit on your legs and back.

7) Create a laser course indoors: Use colored string to create fake laser beams across your home. You can make it more interesting by having a goal to reach. Place an item of jewelry in the kitchen and challenge the kids to get to it quicker than you can without touching the "lasers." You will have to find ways to go over and under the string without touching it! Great fun for all the family.

8) Play Twister: Most families have this classic game somewhere in the garage or the loft and have forgotten what fun it is. If you don't have the game to hand, you can make your own using round paper plates, a sheet, and acrylic paint.

9) Park away from your destination: Even when you must take the car to go somewhere, you will have an opportunity to burn some calories. If you are given the choice park at the far end of the car park as far away as possible, every decision you make helps you become the new you. Twenty extra steps may seem insignificant, but they all add up.

10) Cleaning: We all have to do it; we all know it is dull, so how can cleaning be fun? When you are craving a treat, take that energy, and tackle a domestic challenge. Turn up the volume on the radio and have a soundtrack to your tasks. Vacuuming the carpet can be a real workout if done with vigor! Use all your muscles as you push that bad boy around the carpets. Stairs can be especially challenging, and paying attention to every step will stretch those calve muscles and work the arms. If you want to extend the experience and learn as you clean, try podcasts instead of music. There are some real treats out there, and you can mostly download them for free.

11) Roughhousing: Most of us remember roughhousing with our dads as a real treat. Rolling around in the yard or the living room or being swung around like a monkey. Wrestling and chasing each other felt like the best thing we could do as a family. Unfortunately, our PC world has labeled roughhousing with a bad rap. We are too worried about our kids getting hurt and developing violent tendencies.

The benefits of roughhousing have been overlooked for some time. It has been maligned for too long, and the benefits are obvious. You will help build your child's resilience and teach them how to be adaptable. Throwing your kids will help you form a bond and burn calories.

Of course, if you don't have kids, you can always roughhouse with your partner. Gentle headlocks with a playful partner can soon turn into a different activity, which leads us to…..

12) The horizontal tango: Yep, if you are feeling the need for a snack or a tasty treat, you can replace that type of craving for another. We are not talking about traditional dancing but that special time for consenting adults. A special cuddle can go a long way to burning off your days' calories, and it should be fun! If it's not fun, then you're doing it wrong! And with that, we shall move swiftly on!

13) Martial arts: do you watch Bruce Lee films and think, "I could do that?" well, now is the time to see if you can. There are a couple of ways to use martial arts as a form of exercise. You could just watch any martial arts films and follow the movements on the screen while breaking out in a sweat. Or you can take classes online or at local health centers. The decision is yours; you can keep it simple or take it to the next level.

14) Swimming: Grab your swim gear and head for the beach or local beauty spot. Even splashing about in water will help you get fitter. Water provides its own resistance and makes your body work harder to move. Water aerobics classes are perfect if they are available in your area. If you don't have the luxury of a local beach or lake, then exercise in the bath! Everything counts!

15) Climbing over stuff: If you find walking a bit sedentary, then take your daily stroll somewhere more challenging. Woods and forests will provide you with nature's obstacles. Climb on tree stumps and walk on logs. Leap small streams and climb trees. Nature is awash with outdoor opportunities for climbing.

If you are restricted to more built-up areas, you may want to try Parkour. Leaping buildings and sliding down handrails may seem like a young person's activity, but you can moderate the activity to suit your level of fitness. Begin in your yard with a couple of chairs and a small table to leap before you progress onto bigger things. You can even begin with avoiding cracks in the sidewalk before balancing on the curb.

16) Play kids games: Hopscotch, tag, kick the can all be fun and take you back to your childhood. Hide and seek, blind man's bluff, and even rolling down hills will help you release some energy. Get a few friends to join you and make it even more fun!

17) Become an Ikea guru: Do you need any furniture in your home? Consider a trip to Ikea and the purchase of some classic flat-pack items. You will be lifting stuff, bending, and picking up sections while you build your furniture and hunt for that missing screw. Beware though there may be, no there will be, swearing and cursing! Earmuffs for the rest of the family might be an idea!

18) Have a picnic: We are not suggesting you stop eating altogether, so why not make a regular meal into an opportunity to exercise. Pack a hamper with tasty, nutritious treats and a selection of cold drinks and head for the great outdoors. Spread your blanket, sit down and dig in! You will benefit from all the adjustments in your posture while creating a memorable event for your family. If you can't get outside, then decamp on the living room floor instead.

19) Install a pull-up bar: We all have doorways, so installing a pull-up bar should be simple. Every time you pass through the door hole, perform a pull-up or chin up.

20) Join a club: Fitness is always better when it is a shared experience. You can try adult gymnastics, softball, kickball, or tennis. Rec leagues are a perfect way to meet new people and try new activities.

You may want to do something off the wall and join a LARP club. Live-Action Role-Playing involves reproducing historical battles and other scenarios. Some amazing clubs provide the opportunity to wear costumes, wield weapons, and generally have a ton of fun.

More Traditional Exercising at Home

What if you want to do more regular exercise, but the thought of joining a gym fills you with horror? There are ways to spend a few dollars to bring exercise to you rather than you having to seek it out.

Use Gaming Consoles

Our first option is a little old school. Travel back in time to circa 2006 and Nintendo revealing its revolutionary Wii console. Available with accessories like num-chucks and a balance board Wii consoles offered the opportunity to participate in sports with handheld controllers and a motion sensor, you could take part in interactive games from the comfort of your own home.

Fast forward to 2020, and you can find these consoles available for around $40 or even less online. There are always Wii games to be had at yard sales or online at Amazon or eBay. This can be a great way to start exercising daily without getting bored.

The games available vary in quality. The Super Mario games have great graphics but can involve a lot of practicing to master the movements of the controllers. The platform games and shoot 'em up games are fun but won't involve much movement.

The prime disc for daily exercise should be the classic Wii Sports. The games are simple to understand, and you will be set targets to achieve professional levels of play. You can play tennis, golf, bowling, baseball, and boxing. The boxing is quite lively and needs num-chucks to play.

The tennis can be played against real-life opponents or computer-generated opponents. You can play single games, sets of three or five games, and you score points for your results. Beware, though; you will lose these points when you lose!

Baseball, golf, and boxing also take the same format and gives you an excellent chance to fling yourself around the room. Wii sport is a simple format with good graphics, but it is not overly flashy.

Try your luck on the balance board with winter sports discs. There is also a personal trainer option. If you take the time to set up your personal training program, the online instructor will help you achieve your goals.

If sports are not your thing, then try the dance games. Just Dance has numerous versions to try and will soon have you breaking into a sweat. The catchy routines are normally around 4 minutes long and really test your stamina. The beauty of the dance games is they allow you to concentrate on the one dance and improve or just move on and try another routine.

Of course, the Internet is awash with fitness routines you can follow no matter what your fitness level. You can pay for premium services, but there are excellent free resources to try as well.

Free Online Exercise Resources

1) Fitness Blender: Hosted by husband and wife team Dan and Kelli, there is a host of videos to guide you to fitness heaven! Fat-burning workouts stretch training and kickboxing are just a few examples of the workouts they provide.

2) Sweaty Betty: This may sound like a girl you should avoid, but the online resources they supply are some of the best. They are for all levels of fitness; from gentle yoga to HIIT, they are bound to have something to suit your pace.

3) Jessica Smith TV: This fresh-faced blonde instructor may look like the girl next door, but she is a fitness guru. She offers videos that are 7/10 or 30 minutes long, depending on your stamina levels. Her enthusiastic approach will have burning fat and sweating!

4) Tone it up: If you are simply looking to tone your body and learn some strengthening exercises, then this is the site for you. Let Karena and Katrina guide you through their specific workouts, depending on the area you want to improve. Their style is very personal, and you will soon see results if you commit to their site.

5) Spark People: This site is specifically aimed at people who have limited time to train. They share short instructional videos that make use of your limited spare time. The site is also a great source of nutritional ideas and healthy recipes for you to follow.

6) Diet Health: If you have always dreamed of a personal trainer but don't have the money to spare, then check out Diet Health. Some of the best personal trainers in the US will take time to share their personal exercises and health tips with you. Their workouts are generally under 10 minutes and can be fitted into your busy lifestyle with ease.

7) eFit30: For those of us looking for gentle exercise for people of a certain age, then eFit30 is perfect. They have full-length classes that take a slower pace but still provide a full workout.

8) Gymra: If you are looking for a site that offers an excellent range of workouts, then try Gymra. They offer no equipment routines, dumbbell workouts, absolute beginners, and total body routines.

9) Live Strong: Celebrity trainer Nicky Holender is well known for getting results. This site is filled with online instructions for people who want a quick fix workout that yields results.

10) Steady Health: Designed for people who are recuperating after injury or illness, this site is perfect for those of us that just want to feel relaxed and laid back while exercising. Their easy to follow workouts are designed to get the most reluctant muscles working again.

The bottom line is we all know we can do more exercise, but the examples are given here show us how to achieve it. No excuses now get that body moving!

Part Seven

Lead a Mindful Life

When you turn to food for comfort, it can be difficult to understand why. Our hectic modern lifestyles can make us stressed and highly strung. Food can seem comforting and reassuring, and we use it as a safety blanket.

You may feel that taking thirty minutes a day to meditate is simply unachievable, so how can you possibly practice mindfulness? When your mind is pulled from pillar to post, it can seem that food is your only option for comfort. We are now going to explore some mindfulness exercises that can be practiced anywhere at any time.

Exercises to try when stress and panic threaten to overcome your well-being:

Mindfulness Breathing

This can be done standing up or in a seated position. If you can sit in the lotus position, then great, if not just do it wherever you can.

- Close your eyes and breathe in for 5 seconds. Exhale gently and repeat.

- You should breathe in through your nose and out through the mouth.

- Clear your mind and focus on your breathing.

- Imagine your breath on its journey through your body, filling you with life-giving air.

- Picture your lungs expanding and expelling the air into and out of your body. Follow the path it takes to reach your mouth and see the energy dissipate as you exhale.

If you think you are the kind of person who would never be able to meditate, then guess what? You just took the first step to a calmer, more mindful life!

Mindful Observation

How aware are you of your surroundings? The simple elements that form our world are amazing but can often be overlooked. We can focus on our busy lives and totally miss out on the natural beauty that surrounds us. This simple exercise will help you appreciate nature and the beauty of our natural environment.

- Choose an object to focus on. It can be a flower or a cloud, an insect, or a blade of grass. No matter where you are, there will be something that connects you to nature.

- Relax and study the object. Let the background noises and images fade into oblivion as you concentrate on the details of your chosen object.

- Notice every element that forms the object as if you were seeing it for the first time. Take the time to appreciate colors and textures. How does the object flow and move in its natural environment?

- Connect with the energy that flows around your subject and allow yourself to feel its purpose.

Mindful Awareness

Do you take your body for granted? When was the last time you marveled at your own awesomeness? It's probably been a while! If you want to treat your body with respect and stop binge eating, you need to remind yourself how special you are.

- Choose an action that happens every day. It can be as mundane as you like.

- Once you begin the action, stop for a moment, and be aware of what you are doing.

- Imagine the muscles of your body, working together to perform the chosen task.

- How do you feel? Where does the task lead you? Be mindful of the surroundings and understanding that accompanies your action.

Awareness is not just about physical cues; it can also involve all your senses. When you are listening to music, be aware of how amazing your ears are. They pick up various noises and process them for the brain. Your eyes are amazing too. How do they see things and tell your brain what they are?

Now consider the relationship between your nose and food. The first time you smell food, stop and appreciate what you are experiencing. The aroma of your meal should remind you how lucky you are to share food with family and friends. If you do experience any negative thoughts or cravings, then take a moment to stop, recognize the negativity, and label it as unhelpful. Now discard the negativity and focus on the positive feelings food generates.

Mindful Appreciation

Too often, we sail through life without appreciating how lucky we are. This exercise will help you give thanks for your life and recognize the insignificant details that pass us by.

Pick five things that happen regularly but are unappreciated. For example, the flow of electricity that heats the water for your shower. The clothes you wear to keep you warm. Birdsong in the morning or the sound of children laughing in the park.

Now consider the following:

Why do these things exist, and where do they originate?

- Have you ever considered what the world would be like if they didn't exist?

- How much joy do these processes bring to you and the rest of the world?

- Have you ever considered how all processes are linked and form the functioning of the Earth?

When life seems overwhelming, and stress is dictating your thoughts try one or more of the exercises. You will feel more grounded and aware of your environment. Awareness will help you consider your decisions with a clear mind and a better understanding of consequences.

Now we can try a day full of mindful exercises. It may seem a bit overwhelming at first but stick with it, and you will soon be practicing a mindful lifestyle.

Morning Exercises

Wake Up Early

If your normal morning routine follows the same pattern every day, it may be time to shake things up. If you wake to the alarm, jump out of bed, wash or shower followed by bathroom ablutions, get dressed, grab a quick bite to eat and then leave the house, you are already feeling the pressure as you close the front door!

Set your morning wakeup call 30 minutes earlier than needed. When you open your eyes, take 5 minutes to stretch your limbs and appreciate the quality of sleep you had the previous night. Raise your head and turn to the side. Place your feet on the floor and stretch your arms to the ceiling. Take the time to make your bed in preparation for the night ahead. This will send a signal to your mind that you are prepared for your day and will appreciate the sleep that follows.

Shower meditation is a great way to start the day. As the warm water flows over your body, take time to follow the flow. As your body reacts to the calming effect of the shower, put your mind on autopilot, and allow it to create inspirational ideas.

When you reach the kitchen, take time to appreciate your breakfast and the day ahead. Mentally plan your day and allow time for mindfulness during your schedule. Knowing you will have time to unwind will give you something to look forward to.

As you leave your home, take the time to look in a mirror. Smile at yourself. The first time you do this, there is a chance you will feel ridiculous but stick with it! Smiling slows the heart and relaxes the body. As your smile widens, the endorphins that reduce stress levels will be released into your system.

Take 10 minutes to record your thoughts. Having a handy notebook on the kitchen table will allow you to create morning pages. What did you dream about last night? What were your first thoughts as you woke? What are you looking forward to in the week ahead? Keep your journal upbeat and hopeful. It will become a beacon of hope when times get stressful.

When you are creating your morning, pages set yourself some goals. What are the three things you plan to do today? Why three and not twenty? Three is manageable. The aim is to fulfill your goals and avoid regret. You may well go on and achieve other goals after you have fulfilled the specified three, and that's great! Providing you achieve your goals; everything else is extra.

Now you need to leave the house and begin your daily routine. It may be work, shopping, or taking the kids to school. If your routine involves driving, it is important to recognize how stressful driving can be and how mindfulness needs to be applied.

If you are aware that driving is one of your stress triggers, then change this by completing the following exercise:

When you enter your car, practice mindful breathing for 30 seconds.

- Turn your phone onto silent mode.

- Resist turning the radio on. Maintain silence in the car.

- As you drive away, take note of your surroundings. The road is important, but so are all the other components of your environment.

- As you progress, become aware of your emotions. Are you enjoying the drive, or is it stressful?

- If you get stuck in traffic or someone cuts you up, what do you feel? Acknowledge the emotion, label it, and discard it.

- When you stop at traffic lights, or there is a natural break, practice mindful breathing to calm your mind.

- As you reach your destination, take an extra minute to take deep breaths and regroup.

If you work, it is important to take your mindful practices into the workplace.

Declutter your Space

A visual mess is distracting. Looking for things can be frustrating and lead to stress in the workplace. Once you arrive at work, take a few minutes to declutter your personal space. Decide what to keep and what to throw away. File items that are important for the future but are not relevant today. Consider a desk tidy for your bits and pieces and stow unwanted stationery in your drawers.

Creating a clear, organized space will help you be more creative a productive. It also sends a message to others that you are professional and organized.

Mindfulness at Work

Why do you work? Is it just to pay the bills and feed your family, or do you get satisfaction from your work? Most of us gain some form of satisfaction from our jobs, but it can be easy to lose focus and concentrate on negatives.

Approach your work with a different attitude. Be mindful of the job you do and what you achieve. Take pride in your work and recognize the important part you play in your own destination.

Recognize the effort it takes to do your job and give yourself a mental pat on the back.

How does your workday flow? Are you constantly flitting from one task to another and finding it difficult to concentrate? Try batching your tasks. For instance, if you work with a computer, you will probably need to check emails. What else do you need to do on your work computer? Write reports or fill in time schedules may be, whatever it is, get them done in one batch. Now you can concentrate on work away from your desk. This type of grouping will help you streamline your day and encourage productivity.

Remember to take a break.

Do you ever watch co-workers and wonder how they manage to keep going without taking a break? Look more closely; chances are they are stressed and distracted. Failing to take a break and recharge your batteries does not make you more important or productive. In fact, it does the opposite. Focusing intensely on your work is mentally draining and requires a period of rest to regroup.

Try this mindful technique to help you maintain a presence without burnout:

1) Focus on the task in hand

2) Set a timer on your smartphone for half an hour

3) Work intensely for the set time

4) Take a 5-minute break when the timer goes off

5) Repeat four times and then take a longer break for up to 20minutes or so

Improve Interaction with your Peers

Do you work with people who you like? Do you respect your boss and look forward to your interactions? Sometimes the most challenging part of working is the meld of different personalities that can lead to conflict.

How you behave towards others could be a factor in any work tension. Mindfulness allows us to recognize this fact. There is a mistaken belief that the more aggressive and confrontational you are in the workplace, the more successful you will be. Why not introduce civility, compassion, and kindness into your daily interactions?

Asking a co-worker if there's anything you can do to help is not a sign of weakness. It is a sign of kindness and self-awareness. Be emotionally available and compassionate to your fellow workers and change the work environment.

Exercise at your Desk

If your job is sedentary, it can be detrimental to your health. You can practice your breathing and other mindful exercises while seated, but you also need to move your limbs.

Neck and Head Tilt

Move your neck by lowering your chin to your chest and holding it there for 10 seconds. Expand the exercise by lifting your arms to shoulder length and holding them for 10 seconds. Now tilt your head up and rotate gently for 2 minutes.

Shoulders

While seated, place your arms by your side and bend your knees. Lift your chest and shrug the shoulders as high as possible. Keep the position for 5 seconds and then lower back to the original position. Repeat 12 times. Now expand the exercise with 6 shoulder rolls after each rep.

Torso

Stretching your torso will help you keep supple and relaxed at your desk. Cross your legs and twist your torso in both directions. Place your left hand on your right knee for traction and then swap hands.

You also need to stretch your legs and arms. Take short walks around the office and, if possible, get some fresh air. If you are restricted to indoors, then take a mental walk around your favorite beauty spot. Imagine the sun shining on your face and the smells of nature.

Take a Music Break

If your mind is filled with work detritus, it can be overwhelming. Take a 5-minute break to listen to music and calm your mind, elevate your mood, and regroup your thoughts. When you listen to music, it soothes the mind, providing you choose the right track for you! Try classical music and introduce a new experience to your mind.

Laughter Recess

Remember that smile you gave yourself this morning? Does it feel like the last time you felt happy was at that moment? Life tends to get serious, and we can forget to give ourselves a reason to laugh. Take a laughter recess and transport yourself to a place where you can enjoy a belly laugh. Remember amusing occasions from the past or a silly joke you heard. The Internet is filled with videos that are designed to make you chuckle, so check out the cute cat videos on YouTube.

How to Mindfully End your Day

The transition from work to relaxation can be a tricky one. It can be difficult to forget those emails and projects that need to be addressed. If you fail to mindfully end your workday, you may feel the stress of work following you home. Take ten minutes to finalize your "work thoughts" and ease into your evening routine.

Now you need to take a mini-mental vacation. Even the most successful workday will leave you tired and drained, if not exhausted. You need to leave these feelings behind and transition smoothly into a calmer, more relaxing state of mind.

Take a minute to picture your favorite relaxation spot. Imagine you are at the beach or maybe a sun-dappled forest. This will help you relax and leave stress behind before you move on to the next stage of your day.

Reconnect with your Important Relationships

At the end of the day, it can be tempting to shut out other people, grab your favorite snack, and watch Netflix. Once that snack is finished, it wouldn't hurt to have another, would it? Recognize the scenario? Before you know it, you have binged for over an hour and are now feeling self-remorse.

If you take a mindful decision to change your routine and make meaningful connections, you can remove the temptation to overeat. Reach out with a call or text to people who you haven't seen for a while. A simple "how are you" will open lines of communication and allow you to reconnect. Take charge of your emotional well-being and strengthen relationships with people instead of food.

Give Yourself a Break from Electronics

How often are you checking your devices for updates on social media? Do you feel disconnected if you haven't been on Twitter for the last ten minutes? Well, guess what, the world will still keep turning even if you don't know what your best friend had for dinner! Take a break and give your brain and eyes a rest.

Try more relaxing pursuits. Read a book or do a puzzle. Anything as long as it doesn't involve electronically stimulating your brain. Some adults have found coloring books are a perfect way to wind down after a stressful day. There are even some adult based books available on the market.

Mentally Review your Day

The evening is the perfect time to review the day. What did you do, right? Are there any areas you need to address tomorrow? If you do a thorough review, you can cast the subject aside before you go to sleep. Unresolved issues can haunt our sleep so mindfully deal with them, plan how to resolve them tomorrow, and cast them from your mind. You may benefit from an evening journal similar to the one you use in the morning.

Create a Shutdown Ritual

Use your mindful breathing techniques to prepare yourself for sleep. As you breathe, imagine the different parts of your body relax and fall asleep. Begin at the base of your body and work your way up. Once you have imagined your mind falling asleep, you should be ready to drift into a deep relaxing slumber.

Live Authentically

Once you figure out your needs, and they are met, this step is easy. You have to learn to live a life that is authentic. If your needs are not being met, then you need to focus on communicating these needs. Think of how you can change your life in a way that will help you meet these needs. Also, consider what you can do if the people in your life are not helping you meet your needs.

It can be hard to realize that some of your core needs are not being met in your life. This is especially important when it comes to relationships with other people. If your friends, family, or partner fail to meet your needs, you need to draw some lines. Be honest and focused on communicating your needs.

Forgive Yourself

Once you figure out your needs and make a plan for meeting them, you are on the right path. You will feel more in control and self-assured in your life. However, your past mistakes might hold you back. Don't regret and ponder over what is already done. You have to accept and acknowledge the fact that every person makes mistakes. You need to forgive yourself and just work to improve on those in the future. Your mistakes do not define you. If you think too much about your mistakes, they will prevent you from developing a positive self-view. Give yourself credit for learning your lessons and not repeating those mistakes.

Celebrate Your Quirks

Every person is different in his or her own way. You have to learn to accept your flaws and celebrate your eccentricities. It will help you generate self-love for yourself. Don't focus on what is wrong with you, but instead try to be satisfied with what makes you unique. Don't be embarrassed by your awkward laugh; learn to enjoy it. Even if you have weird teeth, it is okay to smile a big toothy smile. There are things you can improve on; you will find that there are many other things that you should accept and embrace about yourself.

Doing all of this will help you overcome any self-defeating thoughts that bring you down.

Part Eight

Sleep and the Effect it has on your Eating Habits

Consider the times of day when you are most likely to turn to food for comfort. Are they when you first wake up or are, they when you feel fatigued? When you are so tired and drowsy it physically hurts, we can often turn to food to boost our energy levels.

You know the feeling. Your eyes are drooping, the noise levels around you are blurring, and your attention is being drawn to food. Just one quick cupcake will help you get some sugar into your system and reboot your energy, right? Well, we all know what happens next. One cupcake leads to another, and then a quick cookie follows. Once you have reached that level, it is difficult to stop.

So, what if you didn't feel those lulls in energy during the day? What if part of the reason you are succumbing to cravings is that you aren't fully rested? The simple answer to curbing those cravings could be getting a full night of quality sleep. If you spend the day looking forward to snuggling up in bed and then spend hours staring at the ceiling, lets, consider how to change that! Here are some easy and simple adjustments to your routine and environment to improve the quality of your sleep.

The Bedroom

Decoration

This may seem obvious, but have you ever considered how restful your bedroom is? Is it a haven for sleep, or is it a practical environment filled with distractions and clutter? Do you enter your bedroom and immediately feel relaxed, or are you too busy checking your devices and clearing clothes off the bed?

Is your bedroom painted in colors that aid restfulness or is it vibrant and bold? You may have decorated your bedroom to match your personality and chose intense bright tones. Red and yellow may look great, but they can be counterproductive to sleep.

Try choosing a calming tone like blue or grey to mute the energy levels. You can also consider natural colors like earth tones and coral.

Temperature

Sleeping as nature intended doesn't just mean discarding nightwear! It also means adjusting the temperature of your bedroom. We were never meant to sleep in hot bedrooms, so central heat can disturb our cycadean rhythms. The ideal temperature for a bedroom should be around 65 degrees Fahrenheit.

Consider how your internal body clock responds to temperatures as night falls temperatures also lower. This tells our bodies it's time for sleep. If your bedroom is telling your internal clock, it is more like midday as far as the temperature is concerned, then it will resist your efforts to sleep. Similarly, the body doesn't respond to uncomfortably low temperature.

Noise

If you live in a city or a busy neighborhood, noise id inevitable. Even if you live somewhere peaceful and tranquil, you may have a partner that snores or noisy wildlife outside your bedroom window. If noise is responsible for interrupting your sleep, it can make your sleep below par.

There are two simple ways to eliminate noise:

Earplugs

Low-tech but highly efficient. These comfortable plugs can be used at home and away. Amazon has a huge range of stylish options that also include carrying cases and waterproof options.

Noise-Canceling Headphones

If you like your tech and are prepared to spend a few more dollars, check out Amazon for some fancy headphones. Echo has a wireless option that also includes Alcxa and immersive sound options. Sony offers an all dancing all singing option for around $330 that has multiple functions. The bottom line is you can get a pair for around $20, or you can pay a lot more!

There is an alternative way to view noise in the bedroom. Instead of eliminating it, you can introduce soothing sounds. This can be done with a white noise machine. You can use your Google play to create a playlist or buy a specific machine for the bedroom. The Wave

Premium Sleep machine costs around $30 and is simple to program. You can choose a 15-30- or 60-minute option to decide how long you want the machine to play.

Light in the Bedroom

When we sleep, our bodies produce melatonin and serotonin. These hormones regulate various human functions, including sleep appetite, and mood. Low levels of these hormones could be the cause of overeating and cravings.

Any light in the bedroom will affect the production and disrupt sleep patterns. Turn off all devices and draw your curtains completely. Try using a traditional alarm clock instead of a LED device and block any light exposure.

If you are prone to visiting the bathroom during the night, try and avoid turning on the bathroom light. Relieving yourself in the dark will avoid any disruption. If you find it hard to block out any artificial light, try a sleeping mask.

Aromatherapy

So, we have dealt with hearing and sight in the bedroom, but what about smells? Your parasympathetic system plays an important part in your sleep. Essential oils can be used to aid sleep by sprinkling them on the pillow or your bedding. Alternatively, you can put an electric diffuser in your room and choose a calming, restful oil to aid sleep.

The most beneficiary oils include lemon, sage, chamomile, lavender, and bergamot.

Some premixed sleep blend can be used to address particular symptoms like the following:

- Mind and body-calming

- Make me sleepy

- Sleep don't snore

- Sleep with pain relief

- Calm me down

Bedding and Accessories

There is no point in making your bedroom a haven of peace if you then curl up in an uncomfortable bed. Your bed should call to you and welcome you with open arms.

Let's consider the prime elements to make your bed better.

Choose a Good Q0uality Mattress

Having an uncomfortable mattress does not just impact your sleep. It can cause back pain and posture problems. It is imperative to have a mattress that suits your sleep and gives you a comfortable sleep.

If you are already dismissing this option because of the price, then you need to think again. Price isn't always an indicator of quality. Some people prefer soft plush mattresses, while others choose firmer options. You can get a new mattress relatively cheaply, or you can choose a more expensive option. The key is to buy the one that makes you comfortable. Some brands will allow you to test it for a fixed period. Ikea promise that if your mattress isn't perfect, you can return it and choose another one.

If you really can't afford a new mattress, you may want to choose a topper. Mattress toppers offer the option of another layer of support and can turn an uncomfortable, worn mattress into a comfortable base for your body.

Bedding

Sheets are important and can be the difference between a good night's sleep and a great night's sleep. You can choose flannel sheets for winter and satin sheets for summer if you are affected by the temperatures. Soft cuddly sheets made from tee shirt material are great all year round.

Pillows

If you have slept with a pillow that doesn't suit your sleeping position, you know how important a pillow is. Side sleepers need thicker pillows to support the neck and head.

People who sleep on their backs should choose low profile pillows that support the curve of the back.

Stomach sleepers need flat pillows to relieve stress on the neck. High firm pillows will make them sleep in an unnatural position and cause neckache.

Consider the number of pillows you require and what filling is best for you. Feather pillows don't suit everyone, and you may want to consider latex or foam.

Understand the Role Cortisol Plays in Sleeping

Cortisol is a stress hormone that gives us energy. Higher levels early in the day allow us to deal with waking up and facing the world. As the day progresses, we should be lowering levels of cortisol to negligible so we can sleep better. Having a stressful day can trigger too much cortisol production and impede the production of melatonin.

Here are some ways to keep cortisol in check:

- Try mild exercise before bedtime

- Use mindfulness to clear negative thoughts from your mind

- Practice mindful breathing to lower stress levels

- Talk to individuals who make you happy. Toxic people can influence your stress levels, and you can counterbalance this with healthy relationships

- Consider a pet. Pet owners are less likely to suffer from higher stress levels

Consider Radical Changes to your Sleep Patterns

Are you aware that you probably sleep mono-phasically? This simply means that most of your sleep comes in one block of time. If you have traveled to Europe or Latin countries, you may have observed a different attitude to sleep. The afternoon sleep is often known as a siesta, and whole towns and cities empty as the inhabitants take to their beds.

This is known as polyphasic sleep and can be a healthy and natural way to experiment with your normal sleep patterns. Progressive US companies are currently recognizing the benefits of polyphasic sleep and are encouraging the use of nap rooms during the working day.

This type of sleep pattern typically consists of a core sleep at night that is between 5 and 7 hours long and then a nap during the day that lasts around an hour to 90 minutes. This is a biphasic sleep pattern that can be successful if your time restraints allow for it.

There is a school of thought that believes the most effective way of polyphasic sleeping should eventually lead to a core sleep of only 2-4 hours per night. However, when we are using sleep to alter eating habits, this concept may seem a little extreme.

Pre Bedtime Rituals

What To Do and Not Do Right Before Bedtime

How you prepare yourself for sleep will play a major part of your nightly routine. Your lifestyle habits could be the difference between a successful night's sleep and a night filled with restlessness.

Avoid Reading Before Bedtime

How many times have you fallen asleep while holding a book or an e-reader? Probably multiple times. Many of us believe that reading a good book as we drift off to sleep is a great way to promote quality rest. Sleep experts have even said that the perfect way to lull yourself to sleep is with a book.

It may not be true for all people, but for some reading before bedtime is a terrible idea. You will need light to see your book, and we are aware that artificial light prevents melatonin development.

For every example, when you have fallen asleep holding your book, there will be another time when you delay falling asleep with the promise of "just one more chapter," which then leads to three. An exciting and stimulating book can wake your brain up and lead it far from sleeping.

The final reason to avoid reading is the retraining of your brain. The bed should be for two things only. Sleep and sex, the order is completely your choice! Anything else should take place in a different room in the house!

Avoid Intense Movies and TV Shows Before Bedtime

First, it must be stated that a TV set or a device to watch TV is forbidden! You may feel that drifting to sleep while watching the latest episode of your favorite saga is relaxing. In fact, it is far from relaxing. Some screen time is allowed, but try watching nature programs or gentle dramas.

If you decide to catch up on the exploits of the people in Westerns or how the survivors in the Walking Dead are coping, you are definitely going to have your sleep affected! You may love watching the walkers being chopped to pieces by Negan and his cronies, but it is not restful. Horror and action should be restricted to at least two hours before bedtime!

You should also beware of the Netflix binge-watching sessions. Not many of us watch TV in real-time anymore, and the temptation to watch a whole series in one session could lead to a lack of sleep. If you do plan to watch multiple episodes, then plan your evening, so they finish early.

Do Not Exercise for at Least Three Hours Before Bed

Exercise will stimulate you. Your mind and body need to be restful before going to bed, and cardio workouts will cause your cortisol to spike. Another reason is that your body needs to be refueled following exercise, so this means going to bed with food still undigested in your system. A big meal before bedtime also overly stimulates your digestion and prevents natural sleep.

In general, it is not recommended to eat before bed. If you are feeling hungry, then you should have a light snack rather than go to bed hungry. A carb-rich snack will help you stimulate the tryptophan in your system. This amino acid will induce sleep and ensure a good night's rest. Eat something light and under 200 calories to see you through until morning.

Avoid Caffeine, Alcohol, and Water Before Bed

If you have been regularly hydrating through the course of your day, you should be able to avoid too much water before bed. One of the biggest disruptions to sleep can be bathroom breaks. The less liquid you have in your system, the more likely you will sleep through.

Alcohol and caffeine should be avoided as they stimulate the system. The idea that alcohol induces sleep has become outdated.

Bedtime Rituals for a Better Sleep

Draw or Write

Coloring is becoming a popular pastime for adults. We have explored adult coloring books elsewhere in the book, so what about an alternative way of winding down? Simply take a sketch pad, a pencil, and let your imagination loose! Try a self-portrait or a drawing of your pet.

Drawing relaxes you as the simplest art project will help you discard the stressful elements of your day. Be as childish as you like! If you want to draw with wax crayons, then use wax crayons. If you want to do the painting by numbers, then do it! Nobody is judging you. Art is a very personal statement, and you can be as creative as you like.

Journaling

The art of writing is becoming a lost art. We use autocorrect and Grammarly to edit our online content, but when did you actually write something using longhand? Try a daily journal or what about an old-fashioned letter to someone you haven't seen for ages? A handwritten letter received in the post is a joyful occasion. Use a handmade card to make the experience even better!

If you prefer to keep a practical routine in the evening, then you can use your time profitably while writing. Create a to-do list for the next day. List several things you have meant to do and remind yourself for the next day. Sometimes you need a physical reminder for those fiddly little tasks that are forever being overlooked.

Write a gratitude list. We can often become bogged down by negativity and forget just how lucky we are. Write freeform to clear your mind of those niggling anxieties that can prevent quality sleep.

Take a Warm Shower or Bath

If you regularly feel tension before bedtime, a warm bath or shower will help you ease that tension and prepare yourself for bed. Use essential oils to create a calming aroma in your bathroom. Add to the bath or use a diffuser if you are in the shower. Invest in some quality products to enhance the experience. Shower gels and bath products come in a variety of forms and scents, and there are some products designed specially to aid sleep.

Try these popular brands:

Kiehls Lavender Relaxing Bath: One of the best sellers due to its destressing properties. Glycerin, lavender, sea salt and aloe vera ingredients relax your muscles and promote quality sleep.

Vitabath Bath and shower gel: This versatile product can be used in both the bath and shower. It is free from parabens and provides a Zen-like experience to cleanse the soul as well as the body. The sage, green tea, goji, acai, and vitamins all combine to create a relaxing product that appeals to all.

Kiss my Face anti-stress shower gel: This product is made from natural cleansers based on plant-derived ingredients. It is suitable for vegetarians and vegans as it hasn't been tested on animals. The olive oil and aloe cleanse the skin and moisturizes the skin as it relaxes the body.

Set Out What You Need for Tomorrow

Do you wake up in the morning and immediately begin to scrabble around your bedroom? Choosing clothes and getting work stuff together can be a huge distraction. Why don't you take away that stress by selecting your outfit the night before? Have it hanging on your door complete with shoes and accessories you will be wearing?

Similarly, make sure your lunch is packed and ready in the refrigerator. Your work stuff is to hand as well as your car keys if you love a pot of coffee in the morning load the filter, coffee, and water, so you just need to flip a switch.

These rituals will help you to get a better night's rest. As you lay in bed, try visualizing your life in a years' time. What will you have achieved? Where will you be? Drift away with visions of positivity and hope!

Part Nine

Distractions

When you are bored, you tend to reach for a snack to fill the time. This leads to another trip to the kitchen, and before you know it, an hour of binging has passed. Next, there is the sickening guilty feeling that leads to even more eating as you feel your self-esteem shrinking by the minute. Sound familiar? The problem begins with boredom, so what if we replace boredom with something else?

The online world is beckoning you to come off your social media and try something more interesting. If you spend hours on Twitter or Facebook with nothing to show for it, then consider what you could do if you spent your time educating yourself!

Now, before you run screaming from the room with images of the school and boring lessons burned in your mind, think again. There are thousands of educational, interesting, and even profitable courses online. If you don't want the formality of coursework, then try inspirational websites that will help you embrace a new outlook on life.

Courses can be incredibly rewarding in more ways than one. You can gain accreditation that could change your life. Online courses provide the opportunity to change your career, become your own boss, and completely change your life!

Sounds interesting, right? Let's delve a little deeper and see what's out there!

Crafting Sites

Even if you don't consider yourself a "creative type," chances are you can find a course that appeals to you. Some people dismiss crafts as being the type of thing your grandma or spinster aunt would do. This is simply not true. Some of the online crafting sites help you transform your home into a cool, eclectic place filled with quirky pieces you have designed yourself.

Other sites help you learn knitting, macramé, or crocheting. Improve your sewing skills or learn how to dye clothes. The possibilities are endless.

Here are a few courses that may appeal to you:

1) Introduction to 2D Animation for Beginners: 8 different lessons are ranging from basics to finishing touches and takes only 32 minutes to complete. You will be taught techniques that will enable you to draw in 2D, create your own character, and make them wave! The tutor Jack Grayson is extremely easy to follow and will help you understand the basics of storytelling through animation.

2) Creative Writing for All: Acclaimed author Emily Gould offers you the chance to join her and over 20,000 students to take this creative writing 10-day challenge. She provides inspirational examples, revision tips, and is perfect for beginners or enthusiastic writers alike. The course has 6 separate lessons and can be completed in 26 minutes.

3) Isometric Design for Beginners: Isometric design may sound complicated, but it is everywhere! Illustrations to video games this class is designed to introduce you to optimizing your artistic development. The instructor Hayden Aube will take you through the process from fundamentals to Adobe illustrator.

4) Phone Photography for Beginners: We all love taking pictures with our smartphones, but sometimes the results are shocking! We think we are creating awesome memories, but we end up with the back of someone's head or a wonky picture with bad lighting. This course has 28 separate lessons that will take 2hours and 2 minutes to complete. You will learn how to take professional, stylized photos with your phone. Understand all the settings on your phone and learn how to edit with free apps.

5) Discovering Success, Uncover your Purpose, Passion, and Path: If you are unsure where your life is going and what path you are on, then this course is for you. 11 lessons take an hour to complete with different exercises to complete. The host, Emma Gannon, shares her own experiences of the journey from commercial success to her own business, exploring the nexus of creativity and the internet.

6) Stand Out and Make Money on YouTube: If you have always dreamed of being a professional YouTuber, then take this class! Social media personality Jazza, who has over 5 million subscribers, hosts this course that has 15 lessons and takes 2 hours to complete. He teaches you how to work for yourself and create a YouTube channel to promote yourself and grow your own brand. He is brutally honest and explains that it won't be easy, but he gives you all the tools to become successful.

7) The Art of a Side Hustle: If the idea of having multiple income streams appeal to you, then check out this course immediately. Consisting of 18 lessons and takes 49 minutes to complete this class is all about investing in yourself and taking control of your finances. It explains how you can make money on Amazon. It also directs you to the top freelance opportunities available and how to utilize them. The art of a side hustle is one of the best ways to turn your spare time into spare cash!

8) Find Instagram Success: Taking an hour to complete this class has 12 lessons that range from why Instagram is awesome to grow your audience. Taylor Lauren is an acknowledged leader in her field and shares her love of Instagram with her students. She defines the success you can achieve while debunking some common myths about the algorithm. No matter what your level of interest in the platform, everyone can learn from this interesting, informative course.

9) ASL the American Sign Language: If you are interested in signing, then join Able Lingo on this fundamental course. Consisting of 28 lessons, the course takes 2 hours and 35 minutes to complete. Each lesson deals with an individual letter, and students will view the hand signals from multiple angles to ensure precision. The course also included multiple letters and short words.

10) Planning your Life with a Google Calendar: If you have a spare 16 minutes and you want to become super organized, then take this brief 7 lesson course. Google Calendar is a powerful tool, and this course explains how to use it properly. Optimize your time management skills both at home and at work.

All the above courses come complete with downloadable worksheets and other tools you may need. They are all accompanied by a review section, a discussion arena, and a list of resources required. They are succinct, useful, and fun to complete. Try Skillshare.com for hundreds of more courses to distract and educate yourself.

If you prefer to take more career-based courses from accredited universities and companies, there are multiple choices to choose from. Udemy is one of the most recognized sources for online education, but they do require payment. That said, there are always special offers available, and Udemy should not be ruled out purely on financial considerations.

Currently, they are promoting the following courses with accompanying discounts:

Machine Learning A-Z Python &R in Data Science for $13.99 instead of the original cost of $199.99. The course is 299 lectures that cover 42.5 hours. Aimed at all levels of students, the course provides you with entry-level knowledge to IT.

Adobe Photoshop CC for $10.99 instead of the original $99.99. The course is designed to educate you about Photoshop, so you are comfortable creating and designing new projects.

The Ultimate Drawing Course for $10.99 instead of the original price of $149.99. 63 lectures spanning 11 hours of art instruction that teaches the fundamentals of drawing and realistic representation.

Other Sources of Free Courses

Coursera: This online resource offers courses from over 190 leading universities and companies from around the world. The courses are free of charge, but if you want official accreditation, it may involve a small fee. Coursera report that 87% of people who learn from their courses report significant career benefits like promotion, salary increases, or new career paths.

Of course, not all courses are career-based. Here are a few examples of the free courses available on Coursera:

1) Buddhism and Modern Psychology: Hosted by Princeton University, this course offers an insight into the links between Buddhism and science. How the basic claims of Buddha are standing up in the modern world and questions how meditation makes us happier.

2) Healing with the Arts: Offered by the University of Florida, this is a course that gives you the tools to heal yourself with art projects. It delves into physical, mental, and emotional healing along with spiritual wellbeing.

3) Sports and Society: Offered by Duke University, this course studies the role that sport plays in society worldwide. It focuses on popular sports as well as lesser-known ones as it examines the sociology and history of the sport to give you new perspectives on the games we watch and play.

4) Dog Emotion and Cognition: Hosted by Duke University, this course focuses on dog psychology and how they think and feel about humans. The professor shares his insight to help us strengthen the bonds we have with our favorite pets.

5) EDIVET: Do you have what it takes to become a veterinarian? If the world of animal care appeals to you, then take this course hosted by Edinburgh University. It provides taster courses that would be covered in the first year at veterinary college. Experience the study of Veterinary medicine and see if you have what it takes to become a vet.

6) Chinese for Beginners: Hosted by Peking University, this course is aimed at people who are interested in Chinese culture and language. The course teaches basic Mandarin, and students will learn conversational phrases and topics from real-life situations. The course doesn't include the study of Chinese characters and is more designed for enthusiastic beginners.

7) Astronomy Exploring Time and Space: Offered by the University of Arizona, this course is designed for complete beginners with no background in science. Studies include modern astronomy and recent discoveries in space.

8) Stanford Introduction to Food and Health: Offered by Stanford University, this course will help you expand your knowledge of how nutrition impacts your health. You will learn how the impact of high rates of processed foods has increased worldwide levels of obesity and food-related ill-health. The course presents a compelling rationale for a return to simpler times. Home cooking with organic ingredients is just the first step we can take to help the world become a healthier place.

9) What is Contemporary Art? Hosted by the Museum of Modern Art, the course offers an in-depth study of over 70 works of art dating back as far as 1980. It will cover all forms of media, materials, agencies, and power. The course covers traditional art and those made by Artificial Intelligence. You will be invited to accompany artists into their studios and neighborhoods to experience a deeper understanding of how they produce their art.

This course will give you the confidence to appreciate all forms of contemporary art and make connections with your own perceptions.

10) Introduction to Psychology: Hosted by Yale University, this course poses some of the more basic questions that we ask daily. Why are some people racists? What do our dreams mean? What makes us happy? This is a study of the mind and how it works. The perception, decision making, and social behaviors we all encounter are broken down and studied.

All the courses come with an individual breakdown of the benefits the course has provided for others. For instance, how many people got a tangible career benefit or a raise in salary after completion? The courses also provide the syllabus, instructors, reviews, and FAQs that are helpful. They give you an idea of the length of time required to complete the course and are also available in multiple language options.

While some of the courses are free, there can be fees applicable for some. There is an option to apply for financial aid if your circumstances require it.

Coursera also offers the chance to take degrees online. If you missed out on a college education or felt the cost outweighed the benefits now could be the perfect time to gain an official Master's or Bachelor's degree.

The certificates they issue on completion of your studies are all recognized by industry professionals. They could provide you with a new career path simply by distracting you from binge eating.

Guru 99, Alison.com, worldscholarshipforum.com and the Open University are also great places to find online learning opportunities. The internet is a perfect way to find other ways to fill your time rather than sitting on social media with a bag of chips!

What about more fun sites to inspire you?

Of course, you can fill your time with stuff that is fun and will have extraordinarily little to do with your career! The world today is an amazing place filled with information. At just the press of a button, you can find life-changing websites hosted by passionate people who want to share their gifts and outlooks with you. Okay, there are also a load whack jobs who have lost the plot and are posting absolute garbage.

Part of the fun is weeding out the useful from the downright useless. To give you an idea of what you can expect, here are some of the most inspirational sites and some of the world's worst!

Inspiring Sites

1) Duolingo: This site is aimed at people who want to improve their language skills. It is very user friendly and has the format of a game for learning that is addictive! If you love playing games and wouldn't mind learning a new language, then log onto Duolingo now!

2) Fierce Gentlemen: This site is fun for all! It advocates old fashioned qualities that men used to have and how modern men can utilize them in modern times. There is advice for fierce gents and fierce ladies alike. While not particularly cool or ethical, the site considers mixed messages and how they affect us all.

3) Dumb Little Man: If you feel like a chat with an old friend about life's many tribulations, then hop onto this site. Jay White creates this site to furnish you with helpful stuff to improve your life. His informal style makes you relax immediately and follow the flow of this awesome blog site.

4) Fathom: This is a travel website that transports you around the world in seconds. From the first page, you will be filled with an enthusiasm for traveling and exploring. Take mental mini-vacation before you pack your bags and set off.

5) Jamie's Home Cooking Skills: This is one of the best cooking sites online. Jamie Oliver has a passion for food that is infectious. His easy style and cheeky British humor accompany a serious message about nutrition. He has recognized the need for better food understanding and how it impacts health. Learn recipes and tips for creating tasty, healthy food.

Later in this section, you will learn about some common eating disorders that affect people with such irregular eating behavior. Certain criteria help define anorexic or bulimic people, while others are diagnosed with EDNOS or Eating Disorder Not Otherwise

Specified. Most of these disorders have specific and narrow criteria that help different people who suffer and those who don't.

You can differentiate between people with disordered eating and those suffering from eating disorders by using the criteria specified by the American Psychiatric Association. This helps to narrow down the list of people with eating disorders as compared to most others who just have disordered eating.

As you may have understood by now, an eating disorder would be a diagnosis, while disordered eating is more of a descriptive phrase. Despite the superior cause of concern for eating disorders, disordered eating requires attention as well. If someone has unhealthy eating concerns, they need to give it the required attention and treat it before it turns into a more problematic condition.

If disordered eating behaviors are left to continue for too long, they may easily develop into a serious eating disorder that causes severe health problems. Some of the common symptoms of disordered eating are as follows:

- Frequent dieting

- Anxiety-related to certain foods

- Skipping meals frequently

- Chronic fluctuations in weight

- Rigidity in food and exercise routines

- Associating feelings of guilt or shame with eating

- Constant preoccupation with body image, weight, and food

- Compulsive eating habits

- Trying to make up for a bad food binge by fasting, purging, or restricting food.

Most people suffering from disordered eating patterns rarely acknowledge the severity of their condition. They do not realize the impact this behavior has on their body and mind in the long run. Failing to grasp the implications of their habits prevents them from correcting their eating patterns.

Disordered eating can easily increase the risk of eating disorders, obesity, gastrointestinal dysfunction, bone loss, imbalances in electrolytes and fluids, low blood pressure, anxiety, depression, low heart rate, and social isolation. This is why you must realize that disordered eating is a health concern that needs to be taken seriously.

It can be difficult to detect this in some people because everyone does not display the same common symptoms. Keep in mind that someone who has an eating disorder will usually be suffering mentally and physically. People with a history of disordered eating should consider going to a qualified dietician. This will help to treat their condition and improve it instead of progressing towards a serious disorder that can be fatal.

Dieting is a very common form of disordered eating. Studies show that people suffering from serious eating disordered usually indulge in frequent dieting. It is especially dangerous when such people restrict the amount of food they consume.

The metabolic rate of the body is automatically slowed down when it goes into starvation mode. Reducing the rate at which the body burns energy is how it helps to sustain itself when sufficient nutrition is not provided. Such eating restrictions or dieting, in turn, causes them to overeat or develop some binge eating behavior. This is why people who diet too often end up gaining more weight or become obese as well.

When they give up on their diet or indulge in a binge session, it leads to feelings of guilt or failure. They may choose to isolate themselves and stay away from society because they fear judgment or just situations where they will have to eat food. It leads to a lack of confidence and low self-esteem. This is why disordered eating and dieting are considered very dangerous. Dieting is one of the leading causes of the onset of eating disorders. This is why it is important to seek help as early as possible.

Some of the risks associated with disordered eating include:

- Weight gain

- Fatigue

- Lack of proper sleep

- Muscle cramps

- Osteoporosis

- Development of a clinical eating disorder

- Headaches

Thankfully, it is possible to change disordered eating even if it was carried out for a long time. If you get the right treatment and support, it will help in a significant way. It is more important to commit yourself fully to improve your health so that your body and mind can function optimally again.

As we mentioned before, eating disorders are much serious than disordered eating. These conditions result from persistent disordered eating behaviors that negatively affect your mental and physical health.

Eating disorders affect a person's ability to function normally in many areas of life. Most of these disorders involve an excessive focus on body shape, body weight, or food. This excessive obsession leads to dangerous patterns of eating that affect health negatively. Eating disorders also leave a serious impact on the cardiovascular system, bones, digestive system, teeth, and mouth.

If an eating disorder persists for too long, it usually leads to more serious health conditions or diseases. More often than not, these eating disorders will develop when the person is in their adolescent or teen years. However, with the right care, this behavior can be changed and transformed into healthier eating habits.

The following are some of the red flags that usually indicate that a person may be suffering from an eating disorder:

- Frequently skip meals or make excuses to avoid eating food

- Focus obsessively on eating healthy

- Adopt a very restrictive diet

- Excessive and strict exercise routines

- Social withdrawal

- Eating differently from what the whole family or group eats during meals

- Dependence on oral dietary supplements and laxatives

- Constant complaining about gaining weight

- Persistent worry over being fat

- Constantly looking in the mirror and looking for self-perceived flaws

- Eating too much of sugary foods

- Frequent episodes of induced vomiting often accompanied by callused knuckles

- Loss of tooth enamel due to frequent purging

- Frequently going to the toilet during meals

- Showing signs of shame or guilt overeating habits

- Eating food in secret

- Seeming depressed

If you feel like someone you care about is displaying these signs, they may be suffering from an eating disorder. You should contact a doctor in such cases and get them the required help.

Eating disorders may be caused due to genetics and biology or psychological and mental health. However, the exact cause remains unknown. Certain people are at a higher risk of developing an eating disorder compared to others.

Types of Eating Disorders

Anorexia Nervosa

Anorexia or Anorexia Nervosa is a serious and potentially fatal eating disorder that is characterized by extreme weight loss and self-starvation. Some of the common symptoms of anorexia are food restrictions that lead to extremely low body weight in the context of sex, age, physical development, and overall health.

People suffering from anorexia are also known to have an intense fear of gaining weight or becoming fat, which also hints toward other psychosomatic health problems. They have persistent behavior patterns and tics that interfere with the normal process of weight gain, be it through excessive workouts or unhealthy fasting practices.

Anorexia can arise due to disturbing experiences due to body weight or shape, such as bullying, and it is often influenced by a heightened sense of self-evaluation or the inability to recognize the seriousness of your current low body weight. Binge eating followed by excessive "purging" is a commonly observed behavior among people suffering from anorexia.

Depression is one of the most severe medical complications that is closely associated with anorexia. Most of the symptoms of anorexia, such as social withdrawal, insomnia, increased irritability, and diminished interest in sexual activities, also happen to be the early precursors of depression.

Anorexic individuals also tend to develop obsessive-compulsive disorders, both related and unrelated to food. This can severely decrease their quality of life. There is also an elevated risk of suicide if nothing is done to treat it in time. Some of the other dangers that are associated with anorexia are listed below:

- Delayed puberty and lack of development.

- Cardiovascular diseases.

- Hormonal imbalances.

- Heart failure.

- Gastrointestinal problems such as constipation, acid reflux, bloating, and stomach aches.

- Edema.

- Amenorrhea (irregularities in the menstrual cycle).

- Low blood pressure and blood sugar levels.

- Tachycardia (abnormally elevated heart rates) or Bradycardia (abnormally slow heart rates).

- Compromised height and stature.

Bulimia Nervosa

Bulimia nervosa is another fatal eating disorder that is characterized by a cycle of periodic binge eating, followed by compensatory behavioral tics such as self-induced vomiting directed towards compensating for the effects of binge eating.

A regular and frequent binge eating habit is accompanied by an overwhelming sense of loss of control and self-critique. They are likely to engage in regular purging activities and the recurrent use of unhealthy and ineffective compensatory behaviors that are masqueraded as ways to prevent weight gains. These behaviors include misuse or overuse of strong laxatives and diuretics, self-inducing vomiting, unhealthy fasting habits, or excessive exercise. Some of the common risks associated with bulimia are listed below.

- Elevated suicide risk.

- Esophageal injuries (tears and ulcers).

- Infertility.

- Diminished gag reflex and difficulty while swallowing.

- Regular cycles of binge eating and purging every week.

- Amenorrhea (irregularities in the menstrual cycle).

- Gastrointestinal disorders.

- Pancreatitis.

- Callused or scarred fingers.

- Cardiac arrhythmias.

- Dental complications such as extreme tooth sensitivity, dental cavities, bleeding gums, and enamel loss.

- Chronic dehydration and electrolyte imbalances.

- Ophthalmologic disorders such as ruptured blood vessels, cataracts, and detachment of the retina.

- Impaired cognitive functions.

Binge Eating Disorder (BED)

Binge eating disorder is also a serious disorder where the person afflicted will tend to binge eat on recurrent occasions. They consume a large amount of food regularly and have a lack of control when it comes to eating. Episodes of binge eating are usually linked to eating a lot faster than usual, eating too much food even when you are not hungry or eating until you feel uncomfortable.

Binge eaters often prefer to eat in isolation because they are ashamed of how much they eat and have feelings of self-loathing, depression, or guilt after their binge episode. You may be suffering from binge eating disorder if you have a binge session at least once a week or feel distressed about your eating behavior. Unlike in bulimia nervosa, binge eaters don't usually compensate their overeating with any inappropriate behavior like purging.

Some of the risks associated with binge eating disorder are:

- Gaining weight or being obese

- High levels of cholesterol

- Impaired quality of life

- High blood pressure

- Increased risk of heart conditions

- Type II diabetes mellitus

- Risk of gallbladder issues

Avoidant or Restrictive Food Intake Disorder (ARFID)
ARFID is a serious eating disorder where the person faces disturbances in eating and eating patterns, which results in significant loss of weight along with other health issues.

People suffering from this condition usually lose interest in food or even eating their meals in general. They stop eating various foods because of their smells, tastes, etc. They are overly concerned about the negative effects of eating too much of certain foods.

Due to such behavior, people suffering from this eating disorder fail to meet the energy and nutritional needs of their bodies. This results in a significant loss of weight, nutritional deficiencies, psychological issues, and dependence on supplements to meet nutritional needs.

People suffering from ARFID have issues with body image and fail to perceive their body shape or weight healthily. Their behavior is usually characterized as restrictive, choosy, selective, or even perseverant. It has also been seen that they may have some negatively conditioned response to eating, such as vomiting or choking.

Some of the common complications associated with ARFID are as follows:

- Growth slows down

- Significant weight loss

- Emotional difficulties

- Some other complications are similar to those suffered by anorexic people.

Other Specified Feed or Eating Disorder (OSFED)

Most people who fail to meet the criteria of the above-mentioned conditions are usually classified under OSFED. People who have some eating or feeding disorder that causes health issues or impairment in life are diagnosed with OSFED.

They may have symptoms similar to one of the other eating disorders but fail to meet all the criteria required to be diagnosed specifically. This is why they are considered as people with an eating disorder and not just having disordered eating.

The following will help you understand how people are classified under OSFED:

Atypical Anorexia Nervosa

This is when the person meets all the criteria, but their weight is above or within the normal range. If they had significant weight loss, they would be diagnosed with anorexia.

Bulimia Nervosa of Limited Duration or Low Frequency

A patient is diagnosed as such when they meet most of the criteria that fall under Bulimia Nervosa. However, they don't have frequent inappropriate compensatory behavior accompanied by binge eating. They may do this at a much lower frequency than those with Bulimia Nervosa. They may even stop this eating behavior after a certain period, like a few months.

Purging Disorder

People with this condition tend to purge recurrently to try and lose weight or attain a particular body shape.

Night Eating Syndrome

People with this condition have frequent episodes of eating at night. They may either consume excess amounts of food after dinner or even wake up from sleep to eat again. This eating pattern causes the person a lot of distress and impairment in quality of life.

Some of the common problems associated with OSFED are:

- Loss of weight

- Faltering growth rate

- Emotional issues

Unspecified Feeding or Eating Disorder

People with eating disorders that do not fulfill the criteria of other identified disorders are diagnosed with UFED. Their eating behavior causes a lot of distress and affects their normal functioning. Clinicians classify them with UFED if they don't have enough information to mark them under other specific illnesses.

Part Eleven

Create a Structured Day

Think about what triggers your binge eating and the times when you are prone to straying from your healthy regime. Boredom, lack of focus, and low self-esteem can often lead to bad eating habits, so you need to avoid them.

When you wake, it is important to take stock of your life, recognize what the day holds for you, and leave your bed with a feeling of anticipation. Remember the mindfulness attitudes we have already explored and begun your morning ritual with them.

Now it is time to consider food for the first time in your day. At this point, we must recognize intermittent fasting and its health benefits.

Intermittent Fasting

This form of eating is currently one of the most important and popular ways of healthy eating. It works because our bodies are hardwired to eat like this. Leaving gaps of up to 16 hours between meals has proved an effective way of eating healthier. Our ancestors didn't have the option of storing food, so they ate as they hunted and could often go for long periods without food. As a result, humans evolved with the ability to exist without food for longer periods of time.

However, intermittent fasting is not suitable for everyone, and experts recommend that people with eating disorders take a different approach to eat. If you reduce the times you eat, you run the risk of excessive eating due to hunger. People who tend to binge eat are encouraged to eat little and often. Smaller meals regularly are more likely to conquer the disorder.

Breakfast

Forget the fad diets that recommend you skip eating in the morning. You are missing out on the most important part of your daily nutrition. Eating a hearty, healthy breakfast will help you tackle the day with energy and optimism. Make an effort to cook a good breakfast, and your body will thank you for the rest of the morning!

Breakfast Recipes

Smashed Avo and Poached Egg on Toast

Scoop the flesh from a ripe avocado and mash it with a fork. Then Take a toasted piece of whole meal bread and liberally spread the avocado on it. Top with a poached egg and serve immediately with seasoning.

Savory Egg Muffins with Spinach

Take a muffin tray and coat with cooking oil in a bowl mix two raw eggs with fresh spinach and grated cheese. Pour the mixture into the muffin tray and cook for 12 minutes in a medium oven. Serve with roasted tomatoes or peppers for color.

Superfood Smoothie

Take some almond milk and add your favorite berries and seeds. Slice a banana and add to the mixture. Place in a blender and blend until you have the required texture. Add dark chocolate flakes for extra energy.

Yogurt Pot

The evening before takes some tasty Greek yogurt and add fruit and seeds for taste. Place the yogurt in a pot and refrigerate until morning. Sprinkle with chia seeds and consume immediately.

Chicken Omelet

If you have any leftover chicken, you can turn it into a healthy filling for your omelet in the morning. Take two eggs, add spinach, grated cheese, and spring onions before mixing with a fork. At this point, you can add the chicken or leave it to one side. Heat a frying pan with cooking spray and coat with the egg mixture. Cook and serve with the chicken as a filling.

Scrambled Eggs

This breakfast staple can be made even tastier with the addition of tofu and vegetables. Take two eggs, a splash of cream, and add mushrooms, spinach, bell peppers, and spring onion to the mixture. If you want an extra dose of fiber, then add chopped tofu. Cook the mixture in a pan or a microwave and serve with a whole wheat tortilla for a breakfast burrito.

Sweet Potato Toasts

If you are steering clear of bread but miss your toast in the morning, then try these gluten-free alternatives. Preheat the oven to 350F and line a baking sheet with paper. Take a sweet potato and trim the ends. Cut the remaining potato lengthwise to form ¼ inch slices. Arrange ion the baking paper and bake until tender, around 20 minutes should be enough. Leave the slices to cool and prepare your toppings. You can use savory or sweet ingredients to top your" toast" like sliced strawberries or grated cheese.

Once the sweet potato slices have cooled, place them in the toaster and cook until the edges have browned. This may take more than one toasting cycle, so you may prefer to use the grill.

Okay, so now you are filled with healthy carbs, fiber, and fats; it's time to face the world. Of course, your routine will be dictated to by kids, work, and other factors, but the main thing is to fill your hours with interesting and fulfilling activities.

Focus on actions whenever possible. Make time for fun activities at least three times a week and give yourself something to look forward to.

Understand your Danger Zones

Do you normally take the car to a car wash to clean it? Could this lead to a quick coffee and a calorific snack as someone else valets your vehicle? Why don't you take the opportunity to clean your own vehicle? You will be working off calories while saving money.

The satisfaction of a gleaming car and a healthy workout is a great way to spend an hour or so.

When you go for a walk in the park, will you be tempted to pick up a snack from the local deli and eat it on your favorite park bench? Replace that action with a healthier one and consider what else the park offers. When was the last time you flew a kite? It is exhilarating and really good fun! Instead of munching a pastry, try flying a kite or playing Frisbee with a friend.

If you are lucky enough to live near open spaces, you can find loads of activities to keep you occupied. Get back to nature and avoid the temptation to snack. However, if you do see a chance to reward yourself for eating healthier for a week, then don't beat yourself up if you take it! Having a treat is not forbidden; it is simply restricted.

Avoid Cheat Days

Some people feel having time when a certain food is allowed the best way to beat binge eating, but this is not true. If you have a plan to be "good" all week and then cheat on the weekends, you are demonizing certain foods. Your new healthy living regime shouldn't be based on demonization; it is instead fueled by common sense.

Cheat days can lead to gorging on foods simply because you're allowed to. The better option is to allow certain foods to be consumed as a treat when the need or opportunity arrives. You are ideally expanding the range of foods in your diet, not restricting them. If you are craving a sweet snack, then check your local store for fruit and try something exotic you have never tasted before. If you love a savory snack, try the healthy beef jerky that is low in sodium and sugar.

Healthy Lunch Options

You may be lucky enough to eat your lunch at home where you can make tasty meals with fresh ingredients, and that's great. You may even be lucky enough to work near some amazing lunch places where you can choose to eat out every day without jeopardizing your health. However, it may be that for financial reasons or lack of choice, you may need to rely on packed lunches for your midday meal.

This can lead to a lack of nutrition as you pack a boring sandwich, a bag of chips, and a carton of juice for your lunch. This needs to remedy, and the first step is to buy Tupperware! You need a lunch box that inspires you, and this means having the option of packing multiple ingredients without them mixing together and becoming soggy. Choose dishes that have at least three compartments and keep your options fresh and crispy. Try the Addis clip and close boxes for a perfect sized option to put your lunch into. They are small enough to carry yet big enough for a hearty lunch.

Here are some tasty options to make lunch special

All the following options have three separate elements, but feel free to mix and match!

- Cooked salmon on spinach leaves, cream cheese, and pitta bread fingers

- Cooked chicken, couscous and cantaloupe melon slices

- Roasted stuffed pepper, halloumi cheese, and apple slices

- Cooked chicken, sugar snap peas and tomatoes

- Rye crackers, grated cheese, and cucumber slices

- Hummus, carrot sticks and sliced strawberries

- Peanut butter, apple slices, and grapes

- Cooked salmon, wild rice and tomatoes

- Cottage cheese, crackers and two pieces of dark chocolate

- Lettuce leaves, grated cheese, and pesto

- Cooked tuna, mixed salad, and raspberries

- Cottage cheese, spring onions, and cheese crackers.

The possibilities are endless, and you can prep your lunches a couple of days in advance. There is no reason to turn to unhealthy options if you just take the time to plan ahead.

Following lunch, try and get some light exercise to boost your metabolism. Walking or even a quick run works perfectly. Stay hydrated with water, and you will be ready to face the rest of your day with increased levels of energy.

Once the workday has finished, you may be faced with increased levels of pressure to stray from your healthy regime. Colleagues and friends may suggest you stop off for a drink or a snack before you go home. Nobody is suggesting that healthy living means denying yourself a social life, so accept those invitations but keep your resolutions in mind.

We have already discussed the options available to you when eating out, but what can you do if the occasion is just drinking? What if this leads to a night of socializing in a bar, and you are wary of making bad choices? The simple answer is to plan for such occasions. We all know our inhibitions are likely to disappear somewhat when alcohol is included, so how do you avoid slip-ups?

Have a default drink prepared beforehand: You know your triggers. If you love a cold beer, but it then leads to chips and other salty treats, then resists the beer altogether. Try a glass of red wine instead. The wine is designed to be drunk at room temperature so you can sip it. Beer does encourage us to drink it before it goes warm and can lead to gulping! Red wine is less likely to do this, and you can hold onto one glass all evening.

Try a long drink with plenty of ice: If you love a neat scotch or a shot of bourbon, chances are it will be gone in minutes. Replace this option with a long glass of gin and slimline tonic. Pack the glass with ice and a slice to make it last longer.

Avoid cocktails: They may look healthy(ish) with all the fruit and greenery, but the syrups used can boost the calorie content to over

300 per drink. Try a rum and diet coke or vodka and soda for a low-calorie option instead.

Stay away from the bar snacks. Sometimes you can be loading these bad boys into your mouth without realizing it. The bar owners haven't put them there by mistake. These salty flavor bombs are designed to make you thirstier so you can drink more!

So, you have survived a night out with friends and are ready to head home. Walking may seem the healthy option providing it doesn't put temptation in your way. If there are food outlets on your route home, then maybe take a cab instead.

Normal nights won't always include socializing, so what should be your routine on these occasions? Healthy evening meals should be eaten around 6 pm, so they don't interfere with your sleep.

Here are Some Ideas for Healthy Dinners

Vegetable frittata: This glorified omelet makes use of all your leftover bits that are in the fridge. It can be cooked and served immediately or stored and served cold. Cook up a large serving and have it for breakfast or lunch in the following couple of days. Cook any vegetables you are using in a skillet before adding the eggs to avoid a watery frittata. Drain any excess liquid and then add 12 beaten eggs, a cup of sour cream and a cup of grated cheese. Place the skillet in a medium heat oven for 12 minutes until the frittata is puffed with a semi-cooked center. Broil the dish until the top is golden. This dish can also be modified to include salmon, asparagus, bacon, chicken, or ham.

Baked salmon: This simple, tasty dish is exactly what it says! Take a piece of salmon, place it on a piece of foil and season. Add lemon juice or teriyaki sauce for a different taste and close the foil. Place the packet of foil into an oven at 357 degrees while baking for 20 minutes. Remove and serve with vegetables, salad, cauliflower risotto, or any other healthy side dish.

Chicken lettuce wraps: These super healthy wraps are for those people who love their food in one hit! Take crispy lettuce leaves and fill them with cooked chicken, crispy salad, onion, cashews, and sliced bell peppers. Season with salt and pepper or soy sauce and serve immediately.

Instant Pot Recipes

If you love to come home to a meal that is ready as soon as you walk through the door, then consider investing in an instant pot. You simply place the ingredients in the pot before you leave the house, and it is perfectly cooked once you arrive home.

Try These Tasty One-Pot Meals

Chicken Tetrazzini: Brown 4 chicken thighs and add to the instant pot. Add a variety of vegetables and a can of condensed mushroom soup. Add a cup of water, season to taste and leave to cook all day.

BBQ Pulled Pork: Take a boneless joint of pork weighing approx. 4lbs and season with cloves and salt. In the instant pot layer, the bottom with sliced onion. Place the pork on the onions and cover with another sliced onion. Add 2 cups of water to the pot and add chili flakes, garlic, and ginger. Cook all day and then remove the pork from the pot. Shred the meat and return to the juices in the pot. Stir all the ingredients together and then serve with salad and pitta bread.

Chili: Use ground turkey to make the dish healthier. Add kidney beans, tomatoes, chili flakes, and tomato puree to the pot and leave to cook. Serve with salad.

The beauty of the instant pot is it will never overcook your food, and the healthy choices you make in the morning will be available in the evening. This helps you avoid unhealthy choices when faced with the evening meal.

Once the evening meal has been eaten, it's time to chill and let your food digest. Give yourself 30 minutes to reflect on your day. Remind yourself of your mindfulness routine and do any journaling or list-making you need to do.

Now is the time to rid yourself of any negative thoughts. What happened today that upset you or caused you stress? Consider what you could have done differently and how you would cope with the situation if you could travel back in time. Once you have considered everything, then actively put them to one side.

Do One Thing You Love

Now is the time for your hobby or passion. Did you know your brain relaxes when you are doing something you love? You may want to go for a run or work out for 10 minutes. Maybe you want to check up on the online course you are taking and watch the next lesson. Whatever it is you choose to do, make sure it brings you joy.

Now think about who you love to spend time with and take 15 minutes to connect with them. Ring your family or connect with a friend on Zoom. Chatting and laughing will remind you how lucky you are to have these people in your life. Personal connections are important, and sometimes they get neglected because time is running short. Well, life is short; just a quick connection could mean so much to those you have reached out to. Make somebody's day and say hi!

As you prepare for bed, take the time to reflect on what good you have done that day. Every day provides you with an opportunity to be a better person. If you have managed to keep to your routine, then give yourself a mental pat on the back. If you haven't managed to be as good as you would like, then forgive yourself and move on!

Finally, as you brush your teeth and wash before sleep, remember to ignore those pesky bathroom scales. They don't define you. You know how your body feels, and you don't need the scales to confirm or deny your feelings if you do want to know what your weight restricts the weigh-in sessions to once every 14 days. Set a definite day and time and stick to it.

We all have different constraints on our day, but we are all capable of routine. Implementing this type of routine will help you restrict the urge to binge eat.

Keep a Diary for Emotional Eating

In the chapter on what emotional eating is, you may have recognized some of your tendencies and your emotional eating behavior. However, it is important to be specific and identify your emotional eating patterns. Using a food diary is one of the easiest ways to keep track of your eating habits. You will have to write down every instance that you ate, what you ate, what triggered it, and how you felt. When you backtrack on all your meals, you will figure out the instances of emotional eating and be able to tell what triggered it.

Use your food diary to express yourself; however, you want. Recall how you felt before the emotional hunger pang while eating and even how you felt after eating. Noting all this down will help you be more mindful of your responses in the future. You will see that a pattern emerges and that there are particular scenarios that prompt you to indulge in emotional eating. You will also be able to identify the foods that you usually eat in such scenarios.

You will notice that your emotional eating tends to occur when you spend time with certain people. It could be a friend who is overly critical or negative. It could be when you have too much work and are struggling to meet deadlines. It could also be when you have to attend family gatherings that stress you out. Identifying your emotional eating trigger is the first step. Then you can figure out ways in which you can deal with these triggers in a healthier way instead of overeating.

Find Healthier Ways to Feed Your Feelings

You have to deal with your emotions in the right way. If you react to them by eating more food, it will be very difficult to have healthy eating habits. Most of the fad diets you try to lose weight with will also not work. One of the main reasons behind this is that these diets only give you tips that work if you are able to control your eating habits. Someone with no control over their eating patterns will not be able to use any diet to their benefit. They could try going on a juice cleanse but will end up binge eating junk food whenever a stressful situation takes place. Your emotions will cause you to break off from the diet at some point or the other. You cannot keep feeding your feelings with food and expect any healthy changes in your body or mind. If you want to stop this cycle of emotional eating, it is important to figure out other ways that will provide you with emotional fulfillment. It is not enough to only identify your triggers or understand what emotional eating is. From there, you need to find alternatives to negative behavior and do things that will provide you with emotional fulfillment.

Some Alternatives to Emotional Eating

When you are feeling lonely or depressed, call someone who can make you feel better. Confiding in a close friend or just talking to someone you like can alleviate feelings of depression. You could also play with your pet if you have one. They provide unconditional love, and it also gives you a way to be more physically active. You can also take time to look at photos that bring back good memories and help you feel better.

When you feel anxious, find ways to expand this nervous energy. You could go for a walk outside, play with a stress ball, dance to your favorite songs, or just listen to some music.

When you are tired and feel exhausted, indulge in self-care. Drink a cup of tea, light some scented candles, read a nice book, or take a warm bath. You could just sit on the couch with your favorite blanket and watch a movie as well.

When you feel too bored, find something to keep you occupied. Don't wallow in your thoughts, and don't eat. Watch some funny videos, go outside for a walk, meet some friends, or find a hobby. Think of any activity you might enjoy and use your free time to do it. It could be anything from learning an instrument to playing a game.

On the Onset of Cravings, Pause, and Check-In With Yourself

Food cravings usually make emotional eaters feel very powerless. They get a sudden huge urge to eat, and they focus solely on that. It feels like an unbearable urge that has to be satisfied by eating a lot of comfort food. You might have tried to resist these cravings and failed in the past. This makes most people blame their lack of willpower for it. However, in truth, you have a lot of control over your cravings.

Before you have given in to a craving, you need to stop a while and think about it. Don't automatically give in to them and eat mindlessly. Emotional eating causes the person to reach for their comfort food without giving it a thought. Before they know it, half the cake is gone. But if you take a few moments to reflect when a craving hits you, it gives you the chance to make a different choice. Pausing allows you to think and react differently to the situation instead of reaching for food on auto mode.

If you can put off eating for a minute or more, it is a step in the right direction. Don't force yourself to ignore the craving right in the beginning. Just give yourself a few minutes to put off giving in to the urge as soon as it hits you. The more restrictive you are with yourself, the more you may want to give in. So start slow by just telling yourself to pause for a while before eating. During this time, you should check in with yourself. Pay attention to how you are feeling and what emotions you are experiencing. When you become more aware of it, you will be able to understand why you were eating. It will help you identify triggers and prepare yourself to deal with it better the next time you face a similar situation.

Accept All Your Feelings, Bad and Good

Emotional eating does not stem from being powerless over food. It is caused by your lack of control over your emotions and your response to them. You probably find it easier to avoid troubling emotions by eating food instead of dealing with the feelings. It can be admittedly uncomfortable to confront some emotions. It might make you feel powerless and that it will cause a bigger problem if you face those emotions. However, you should not be suppressing them or even obsessing over them. If you don't do this, then your feelings will eventually pass. No matter how difficult or painful those emotions may seem at the moment, they eventually subside. They will not have lasting control over you if you don't let them. If you push them down or overthink them too much, it affects you more negatively. They tend to build up and fester inside you. Instead of letting it out, you are just adding to your problems by eating more. You have to become more mindful and learn how to connect to each moment as it passes. It will help you to rein in stress, and you will be able to repair emotional issues that usually trigger emotional eating for you.

Indulge in Food without Overeating

Stop eating to feed your feelings. Emotional eating causes you to eat quickly in a mindless way. You just keep eating without a thought and with complete disregard for taste or anything. You don't even realize how much you have eaten till you start feeling physically uncomfortable. It causes you to miss out on the taste or texture of your food. Since it is not physical hunger, there are no cues to tell you have you have eaten enough either. However, if you start eating slowly, it will help you savor every bite you take. You will enjoy the food you eat a lot more and be less likely to eat more than you need.

You can indulge in your favorite foods without overeating them. You have to learn how to savor what you eat. Instead of taking big bites and swallowing it down, take small bites and chew well. It will allow you to have a better experience with your food. Mindful eating is healthy and is completely different from emotional eating, which is mindless.

You have to focus on your experience of eating. Take time to eat each bite and put your spoon down at times. You don't have to be on autopilot and keep putting food into your mouth as soon as you gulp down a bite. Different foods have different smells, textures, tastes, and colors. Mindful eating allows you to experience all of it. You are able to tell how the food really tastes when you take a bite. When you eat slowly, you can appreciate every bite of food. You will feel full much sooner and won't end up overeating.

Mindful eating allows you to indulge in your comfort food without feeling guilty or shameful because you won't be overeating like you usually do. The body takes time to send signals to the brain when the stomach is satisfied. If you keep gulping down food without stopping, you end up eating much more than you need. Take time between bites, so you get the chance to learn how much is enough for you. Your hunger will be satiated this way, and you will avoid eating more than necessary. People who eat fast and chew less are much more likely to gain weight as compared to those who eat slowly and mindfully. It is also important that you focus solely on eating during a meal. Don't eat when you are driving or working. Avoid eating in front of the TV as well. This distracts you from the food, and you keep eating even when you are not hungry anymore. It prevents you from enjoying your meal and does not leave you feeling satisfied.

Use Healthy Lifestyle Habits to Support Yourself

Physical and mental wellbeing is crucial for every person. When a person is physically healthy, gets sufficient sleep, and rest and is mentally strong, they are able to handle any problem that life throws at them. However, if a person is weak and exhausted, the smallest problem can seem like a big issue for them. It sets them off, and for emotional eaters, it sends them directly in the direction of food. If you get restful sleep, exercise often, and lead a healthy lifestyle, you will be able to deal with any stressful situation without indulging in emotional eating.

It is important to exercise on a daily basis. It does not have to be some high-intensity workout that you don't enjoy. Physical activity can be carried out in many different ways. Getting a little exercise every day is actually much easier than most people assume. You could go for a walk or a run, take a swim, get on your bike, or even try yoga. All of these will do wonders for improving your mood and increase energy levels. Exercise is also a great way to reduce stress and helps you think more clearly.

Try to get sufficient sleep every night. Aim for eight hours on a daily basis. Lack of sufficient sleep often causes cravings in the body. It makes you reach out for sweets and other unhealthy foods since they provide a fast boost of energy. If you are rested and get enough sleep, you will have better control over your appetite and cravings will be reduced.

Take time to relax every day. Set aside some time to relax and unwind every day. Try to do this for at least fifteen to thirty minutes regularly. You can just lie down and close your eyes for a while. You could also try meditation. Use this time to just focus on yourself and forget any other responsibility or trouble you may be facing. It will be like a time for recharging your batteries so you can function optimally again.

Connect with people. Don't cut yourself off from people. Connections with others play an important role in your wellbeing. Put in the effort into your close relationships. Make time to take part in social activities. Surround yourself with people who support and encourage you. Spend more time with people who are positive and improve your mood every time you see them.

The following are some general tips that will help you in your struggle with emotional eating.

Tips to Help Overcome Emotional Eating

Look at how you eat. It is more important to take notice of the way you eat than what foods you eat. The specific foods that you choose to eat play a smaller role compared to the amount of food you consume, your eating habits, attitude towards food, and the way you balance your meals. You have to take the time to look at all of these things separately and analyze your eating patterns. It is important to learn the difference between emotional eating and normal eating. You have to implement self-help strategies that will help you address your relationship with food. You need to learn how to say no to the foods that harm your body. You also have to exert more control over the way you eat, so you make better choices. It is important to deal with emotionally charged situations in a healthy way instead of turning towards food to cope with the situation.

Pay Attention to Signs of Addictive Behavior

Many studies have been conducted over the years to understand the relationship some people have with food. The food itself is not addictive, but the person's behavior towards food can be addictive. Some such behaviors include preoccupation with food, losing control, gaining temporary satisfaction from food, and getting ill or gaining weight due to overconsumption. It is important to recognize patterns of such behavior.

Hunger Cues are Different From Emotional Cues

It is important to identify the difference between these two types of hunger. However, it is not always easy to understand if you are physically hungry or just reacting to some emotion and turning towards food. This is why it is important that you learn how to separate the two and regulate yourself. Mindful eating will help you to eat in a healthy way. You have to pay attention to physical hunger signals and push away emotional triggers. Emotions should be dealt with in the appropriate way and not with food. Think of your hunger in terms of ratings. If you are at a five or above, you can eat. If you are only at two or three, control yourself till you are really hungry. However, you should not avoid eating until the point that you end up overeating in response to extreme hunger.

Create a Schedule for Yourself

Eating meals on time is a very healthy habit. Schedule your meals and eat them on the designated timings. Schedule time for snacks as well so that you avoid eating randomly or overeating. Random eating will only cause you to eat more than you need. It is recommended that everyone should eat three main meals and two small snacks in between. Food takes some time to digest after a meal, so you won't be really hungry till after an hour or two after your meal. At this point, you can schedule a small snack that will sustain you till the next meal. It is important not to overeat snacks since it prevents you from eating healthy food during your mealtimes.

Adjust Your Eating Patterns

Eating patterns play an important role. People who have irregular and unhealthy eating patterns tend to gain extra weight. So avoid skipping meals, especially breakfast. Exert some self-control and avoid any midnight snacks or late-night meals. You have to pay attention to the eating routine that you currently follow and acknowledge what is unhealthy. Adjust your pattern according to what works best for you and what will help you eat in a better and more mindful way.

Find Balance

You have to find your balance with everything in life. This will allow you to be satisfied with most aspects of your life. Pay attention to your emotional, spiritual, and physical needs, and try to keep it all balanced. This concept of balance applies to food, as well. You don't have to cut off all your favorite foods just to lose weight. But you should be eating more healthy foods and less of these unhealthy foods. If you eat too much junk food instead of fresh fruit and vegetables, it will automatically affect your body and mind. The physical balance is lost, and it makes you gain weight and become more lethargic. It also makes you dependent on the temporary satisfaction that such foods provide. Work on balancing out your food habits and also try to find balance in other aspects of your life. All of it is connected to each other and makes a difference to your pattern of emotional eating.

Use Healthy Behavior as a Substitution

You may have noticed that you react to emotional situations by eating in response. Now you have to consider what you can do to change this. Think of various activities that don't involve food. You have to substitute your response with one of these activities instead of turning towards food. One of the simplest and most helpful things to do would be to go on a walk. It could be regular walking or even walking on a treadmill. If you have a dog, take it out for a walk. You could try other activities that you enjoy, such as painting, knitting, or anything that gives you something physical to do. It will also help stimulate your creativity and prevent you from wallowing in your emotions. If you can substitute your emotional eating with something more pleasurable or productive, you will find it easier to stop overeating.

Take Support

You don't have to do it all alone and feel burdened. A support network plays an important role in the path to recovery. You could turn towards your family, friends, or even some professional like a therapist. They will play a crucial role in keeping you motivated and encouraged. The people who care about you will cheer on your efforts and also help you along the way with small things like healthier recipes. They will help you deal with any overwhelming emotions and help diffuse the situation. They can also give you company when you go for walks or exercise in any way. Turn to them for help instead of counting on food to make you feel better. A good support system helps people in a big way.

Believe in yourself. More than anything, you have to have self-belief and self-confidence. Motivate yourself all the time and trust that you will reach your goals. Don't set unrealistic goals of being successful and happy all the time. Just learn to deal with all your problems in a better way and focus on your successes instead of your failures. Push yourself to do better in small ways every day. Don't be defeated by small setbacks because you can always get back up and running.

While a support system is important, your relationship with yourself is even more important. Turn to self-validation and don't seek approval from others. Do what is best for you.

Conclusion

You now have the tools to conquer your demons. BED has been with you for a long time, but now it's time to break away from it. Your new regime is all about a healthier you and ditching bad eating. This doesn't mean you need to have a boring diet, quite the opposite, really. You have a new understanding of how food works. You know what your body needs and why. Food should be a source of joy rather than stress.

Binge Eating Disorder has been your primary relationship for way too long. Break those ties, set your body free, and good luck with your new life.

Resources

http://www.naishanks.com

http://www.pocketmindfulness.com

http://www.psychologytoday.com

http://www.eatingwell.com

http://www.hydration.com

http://www.eatthis.com

http://www.healthline.com

http://www.sleepadvisor.com

http://www.livescience.com

http://www.greatist.com

http://www.webmd.com

http://www.nerrdfitness.com

http://www.futurelearn.com

http://www.coursera.com

http://www.lifehack.com

http://www.edit.co